WHAT IS LIFE? WHAT IS HAPPINESS?

BOOKS BY ALLA P. GAKUBA, BSCE, MAS, PhD

Trilogy: motivational nonfiction short stories
to teach logic, creativity, new skills, and
self-esteem that would change readers lives:

What Is Life? What Is Happiness?
(Book 1)

*A Person Is a Product of Time, Place,
and Circumstances*
(Book 2)

*How to Design Innovations and Solve
Business and Personal Problems*
(Book 3)

Alla P. Gakuba, BSCE, MAS, PhD

WHAT IS LIFE? WHAT IS HAPPINESS?

Book 1 in the trilogy: motivational nonfiction short stories to teach logic, creativity, new skills, and self-esteem that would change readers lives

Copyright © 2015 by Alla P. Gakuba, BSCE, MAS, PhD
All rights reserved.
Library of Congress Catalogue-in-Publication Data
Gakuba, Alla P., BSCE, MAS, PhD
What Is Life? What Is Happiness? Book 1 in the trilogy: motivational nonfiction short stories to teach logic, creativity, new skills, and self-esteem that would change readers lives / Alla P. Gakuba, BSCE, MAS, PhD. First edition.

pages cm
Published by Knowhow Skills, San Francisco Bay,
California, USA;
www.allapgakuba.com

Hardcover: ISBN 978-1-943131-04-4
Paperback: ISBN 978-1-943131-00-6
Kindle: ISBN 978-1-943131-01-3
PDF: ISBN 978-1-943131-02-0
EPUB: ISBN 978-1-943131-03-7

LCCN: 2015901018
1. Self-Help – Personal Growth – General. 2. Self-Help – Motivational. 3. Self-Help – Happiness. I. Title.
KEYWORDS: 1. Motivational stories. 2. Happiness. 3. East Africa. 4. General health. 5. World War II.

First Edition 2015

Book designed by Marian Oprea

Printed in the United States of America

10 9 8 7 6 5 4 3 2 1

To my grandsons Paris and Apollo,

with expectations that they will grow into fine men of dignity and honor who will not live selfish lives, but instead will have a purpose in life and make contributions to society, the country, and the world.

TABLE OF CONTENTS

ABOUT AUTHOR	1
PREFACE	5
A GUIDE TO READING THIS BOOK	9

SHORT STORY #1
WHAT IS LIFE? OR, NIGHTS OF CABIRIA — 13

SHORT STORY #2
WHAT IS QUALITY OF LIFE? OR, A CONVERSATION BETWEEN AN EAGLE AND A SNAKE — 21

SHORT STORY #3
A FOOL AND A COMMON SENSE. OR, 5 DONUTS AND 1 BAGEL — 31

SHORT STORY #4
THERE IS NO ROYAL ROAD TO KNOWLEDGE. OR, A LESSON FROM ALEXANDER THE GREAT — 37

SHORT STORY #5
EVERYONE HAS THE SAME AMOUNT OF ENERGY; IT ALL DEPENDS WHERE YOU PUT OR CHANNEL IT — 43

SHORT STORY #6
OUR MIND IS A TAPE RECORDER — 52

SHORT STORY #7
WHAT IS HAPPINESS? OR, WHAT WERE THE HAPPIEST YEARS OF YOUR LIFE? — 62

SHORT STORY #8
AFRICA: AN INTERRUPTED DREAM OR, WONDERFUL LIFE DISCOVERIES IN UGANDA, RWANDA, KENYA, AND TANZANIA — 105

TABLE OF CONTENTS

SHORT STORY #9
PASSION. BELIEVE IN YOURSELF AND
ACHIEVE YOUR DREAMS. AN UNEXPLAINED
PHENOMENON ... 120

SHORT STORY #10
WHY DO AFRICANS HAVE LESS HEART DISEASE,
DIABETES, AND CANCER? AND NO DEPRESSION,
OSTEOPOROSIS, ARTHRITIS, OR ASTHMA? ... 128

SHORT STORY #11
HONEY IS A MEDICINE ... 142

SHORT STORY #12
AFRICA: PAST, PRESENT, AND FUTURE ... 148

SHORT STORY #13
WHAT WAS WORLD WAR II? WHO WON
WORLD WAR II? WHAT WAS THE GREAT
PATRIOTIC WAR? ... 157

SHORT STORY #14
COWARDS. OR, BLOOD IS THICKER
THAN WATER ... 186

SHORT STORY #15
NO MONEY, NO FUNNY.
OR, FROM RENTERS TO HOMEOWNERS ... 198

SHORT STORY #16
WHO ARE YOU? ... 208

SHORT STORY #17
WHO IS MORE INTELLIGENT?
A PERSON OR A COMPUTER? ... 215

SHORT STORY #18
MY 2-YEAR-OLD GRANDSON PARIS' WORLD ... 224

TABLE OF CONTENTS

SHORT STORY #19
WHAT IS A LIFE SPAN?
WHY MAN-MADE THINGS DEPRECIATE AND NOT
APPRECIATE? 232

SHORT STORY #20
ONLY ONE THING IN LIFE IS
CONSTANT—CHANGE. OR, RISE, FALL, AND
DISAPPEARANCE OF EMPIRES AND POWERFUL
COUNTRIES 243

ACKNOWLEDGEMENTS 257

ILLUSTRATION CREDITS 259

THE AUTHOR'S, ALLA P. GAKUBA, BSCE, MAS, PhD,
CONTRIBUTIONS TO ENGINEERING,
TO NATIONAL WEALTH, AND TO WOMEN:
The Forces of Innovation…Conflict? 263

HAVE YOU READ? BOOKS BY
ALLA P. GAKUBA, BSCE, MAS, PhD 269

ABOUT AUTHOR
□ □ □

When attending civil engineering university in her native city Odessa, on the Black Sea, the Soviet Union, the author, Alla P. Gakuba lived an ordinary life. She was a shy, timid, and unsure of herself young woman, but a serious student.

Fascinated with life, bubbled with infinite youth energy, and curious about the world, she had read hundreds classic books written by world famous classical writers.

She saw numerous movies, the majority of them international, and went to the theater many times to hear the most popular operas, saw ballet performances, not to mention visits to the drama theatre, the circuses, and philharmonic classical music performances, all from a young age.

She was a dreamer…In her dreams she was anything she wanted to be. Intoxicated by life she imitated her heroes and adopted their manner, language, attitudes, and became as sophisticated as they were.

Then, one cold, unassuming November evening, fate suddenly interfered and changed her destiny. Fate propelled her to live on different continents, ambushed her with

ABOUT AUTHOR

life-threatening events and monumental problems.[1] She survived, became stoic, and make many contributions.

Alla worked in 4 countries: the Soviet Union, Rwanda, Tanzania, and the United States; in 3 languages: Russian, French, and English; and under 2 radical systems: socialism and capitalism.

Alla P. Gakuba, received her BSCE from Odessa Civil Engineering University in the Soviet Union; she earned her master's degree at Johns Hopkins University, Baltimore; and she received her PhD from George Washington University, Washington, D.C.

Some of Alla P. Gakuba's, BSCE, MAS, PhD, contributions:
- She designed alone, one person, a 10-span bridge with 4 ramps, I–95, in downtown Baltimore, over the Patapsco River.

- She found the solution how to design "a spiral" and then designed it for 3.5 miles of the Baltimore subway aerial structure which is considered to be the most challenging engineering design.

- She was the 1st woman to receive a PhD in the Management of Science, Technology, and Innovations field.

- Her dissertation is considered to be in the top 5% among 250–300 dissertations written in the last 15 years.

ABOUT AUTHOR

- In health care, Alla P. Gakuba created several innovations. One of her innovations sparked an entirely new industry. It created hundreds of thousands of new jobs. As it grew, it started bringing millions, and then billions, of dollars yearly in new revenue to many companies.

- Please see more author's contributions at the end of this book. Alla P. Gakuba's contributions to engineering, to national wealth, and to women: *The Forces of Innovation... Conflict?* by Carissa Giblin, article provided by the Society of Women Engineers, *The Florida Engineering Journal, January 2004.*

---

[1] About Alla P. Gakuba's life-threatening events and monumental problems please read her short story # 7: "What Is Happiness? Or, What Were the Happiest Years of Your Life?" in Book 1 (the trilogy): *What is Life? What is Happiness?*

PREFACE

□ □ □

My intention is noble. It is my obligation to write this book to share and pass on to other people—and especially to younger generations—my wisdom, information, knowledge, creativity, and skills that I learned and accumulated by working and living on 3 different continents, working in the engineering profession, learning from my extensive education, reading numerous books, seeing plays and movies, meeting and working with hundreds of people of different nationalities, gleaning knowledge from mentors, experiencing life-threatening events, facing monumental problems, and from living in several countries and visited many.

I took some inspiration for my book from ancient Greek mythology, which taught people wisdom, new skills, and common sense by using conversations between gods or between animals. The analogy to ancient Greek idea in this book is illustrated in a short story about quality of life "What is Quality of Life? Or, a Conversation Between an Eagle and a Snake."

The book has many *Laws of Life* stories: "There Is no Royal Road to Knowledge," "What Was World War II?", "Who Is More Intelligent? A Person or a Computer?", "Honey Is a Medicine", "What Is a Life Span?", and many more.

PREFACE

Another story titled "Everyone Has the Same Amount of Energy; It All Depends Where You Put or Channel It." And where are the younger generations channeling their energy today? They have "doped" their brains 24/7 on social media (Facebook, Twitter, e-mail, blogs), apps, texting, Disney World fantasies, *Dancing with the Stars*, hip-hop music, and the Kardashians. Yet, at the same time, they have remained oblivious to the outside world.

"Our Mind is a Tape Recorder" is another of the *Laws of Life* stories. Our mind records everything that it hears, sees and reads. Information from texting and social media is not the real knowledge a person needs to have in his or her brain storage.

Fate. If someone before asked me to write a fiction essay on what my life could be, in my wildest imagination I could never compose such a thriller as my nonfiction life soon became.

When attending civil engineering university, I was young, shy, and timid. I had a low self-esteem, but I was hardworking and serious student. Little did I know that fate had a different plan for me. Suddenly, destiny interfered—it made my life a thriller—and propelled me to work on 3 different continents: Eurasia, Africa, and North America.

Fate ambushed me with many life-threatening events and impossible challenges. Then, for all my sufferings, it remunerated me with unique opportunities and wonders—I became strong, fearless, and creative, and began believing in myself.

Some of these life-threatening events and opportunities are described in several *Laws of Life* stories, one of which is titled "What Is Happiness? What Were the Best Years in Your Life?"

Life is full of surprises, both big and small unexpected stressful events. They are occurring many times a day and every day. These events challenge people's knowledge, creativity, and skills and test their endurance, resilience, and ability to survive.

Experiencing a problem? Having difficulties? Overwhelmed or stressed out from life? "C'est la vie!" That's life. What else do you expect? (This for the French is a typical answer.)

That is why from the beginning of civilization to the present time, humans propensity and quest were to find happiness—that is, to find those rare moments to sprinkle life's difficult events with happiness.

This book is motivational and inspirational, is full of ideas, new skills and discoveries about life, happiness, where to channel your energy, how to believe in yourself, find out who you are, and much more.

I challenge my readers to engage, learn, and think. That is, to add to their brain's database real skills and information which they learn in this book. So they can become knowledgeable and sophisticated and have no difficulties in solving life's challenging problems and confront stressful events.

Alla P. Gakuba, BSCE, MAS, PhD
San Francisco Bay, California, USA

A GUIDE TO READING THIS BOOK

□ □ □

This is a book 1 in the trilogy[1] of motivational nonfiction short stories to teach logic, creativity, new skills, and self-esteem that would change readers lives.

It consists of 20 nonfiction know-how short stories.

Readers have 2 options when reading these stories. The 1st option is to read them in sequential order (i.e. one story after another). The 2nd option is to scan the Table of Contents and choose which story to read 1st.

Readers will notice short, repetitive facts in some of the stories. That was done intentionally to ease the flow of reading, instead of referring readers to different stories for facts.

At the end of each story, there is a summary—*The moral of the story*—which states what that particular story is teaches and what questions it answers.

---

[1] Book 2 in the trilogy: *A Person Is a Product of Time, Place, and Circumstances*. Book 3 in the trilogy: *How to Design Innovations and Solve Business and Personal Problems*.

WHAT IS LIFE? WHAT IS HAPPINESS?

SHORT STORY

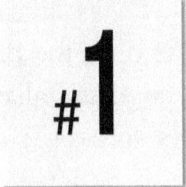

WHAT IS LIFE?
OR, NIGHTS OF CABIRIA

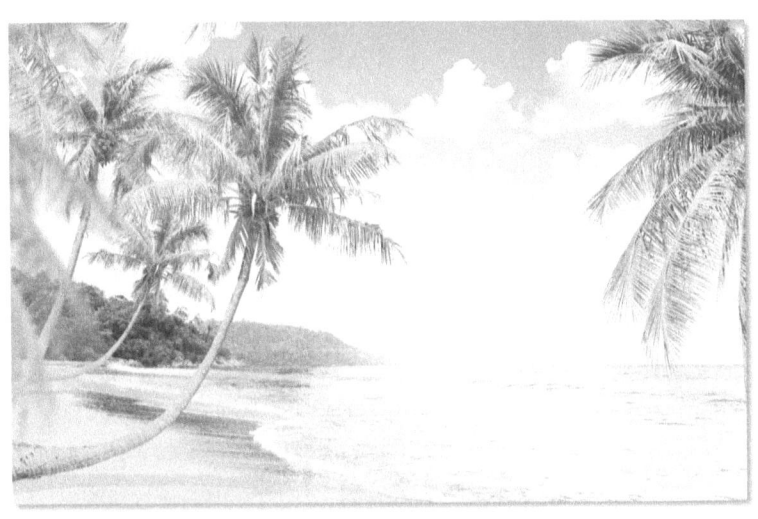

◻ ◻ ◻

One late spring, when I was an engineering student in my native town of Odessa on the Black Sea in the former Soviet Union, a very popular Italian movie was running in many movie theaters across the city. Most of the local population went to see it, waiting for hours in lines that stretched around several blocks.

It was an Italian movie by famous filmmaker Federico Fellini, adored by many Russians. Cabiria, a young woman and prostitute, was a major character in the movie and was played by famous actress Giulietta Masina. The Russians loved and admired her.

I knew the story well; the movie was the talk of the town. I did not go to see it. I was young, idealistic, and was not interested in such a movie. Until one of my best friends, Rita, asked me, "Did you see *Nights of Cabiria?*"

"No," I answered firmly. "What was there to see? The life of a prostitute?"

"Oh, no, no! Do not say that!" my friend rejected my harsh verdict. "The movie is not about a prostitute. It is about life! I have already seen it 2 times!" Her body wobbled with emotion, her voice cracked, and her eyes filled with tears. She clung to my arm and declared, "Let's go! Let's go!" and escorted me to the movie theater. We went in.

WHAT IS LIFE? WHAT IS HAPPINESS?

Rita's emotions, like a thick fog, lingered with me. I saw the movie through her eyes.

The movie started with a short episode. A projector scanned a wild beach populated by endless dunes, where a poor fishing village was located. Representing the village were small, single story dwellings, dilapidated by weather, disrepair and age, scattered unassumingly between the dunes.

At the end of the village near a small crowd of people, there was some commotion on the beach. As the camera moved closer and brought the commotion into focus, it revealed that the beachgoers were actually attempting to revive a middle-aged woman who had drowned in the nearby sea. Some men held the woman's body upside down by her feet, shaking her in order to extract sea water from her body through her mouth, nose, and ears.

One onlooker in the crowd was a young woman. Dressed in a summer cotton dress and barefoot, she watched the reviving action with great emotion. When the rescuers exhausted all their attempts to revive the woman, they carefully lowered her lifeless body and stretched it out to full length on the sand.

The young woman, disappointed and saddened by the woman's death, removed herself from the crowd, and, somewhat unsure of herself, started walking slowly towards the village. There, in the middle of a line of small dwellings, stood her small, single story, dilapidated shack. It was her home, a roof over her head, the place where she grew up throughout her childhood. After her mother died, it became her home and her only asset and possession.

Her name was Cabiria. She had no job. There was no job for her in that poor fishing village, lost among dunes and wild beaches. How was Cabiria able to support herself? The movie revealed the answer. She worked at nights in one of the oldest women's professions—prostitution.

Then one day, she had a breakthrough. She met a young man, one of her clients. He was completely different from all her previous clients. For a change, he took a keen interest in her, asking about her life, and treating her as though she was someone very special.

Quickly, she fell in love with him. They started planning their new life together. He encouraged her to sell her small house, so they could move to a big city, far away from the village and her past. Excited, she sold her home.

They took a train and headed to the big city. In the train compartment, Cabiria was seated next to a big window. Beaming with happiness, she was grateful for her good luck. From the train window, she watched how with every minute she was distanced from her old life and was headed toward a new life.

Ahead was a new dignifying life with the man she was madly in love with, along with new places, people, and new beginnings. It felt like a dream. The speeding train's whistles, boarding and leaving crowds, and the passing small towns and stations all reinforced that she was not dreaming.

Abruptly, at one stop, she got a fright as an electrical current-like sensation twisted her body. What was wrong? Her intuition alerted her to immediate danger and brought her back from her dreams to reality.

Looking for reassurance, she turned her head, expecting to see her lover next to her. His seat was empty. He was gone, along with the money she had received from selling her mom's home.

In disbelief, Cabiria whispered to herself, "Is it true?" The metal friction of the moving train wagons and the accelerating speed and whistles of the departing train answered her question.

Shocked by her lover's betrayal and abandonment, her mind began racing; short-circling, searched for a simple, quick solution. Soon, it found the solution and she agreed with it.

Now she knew how to stop her feelings of despair and agony: the same way that middle-aged woman who recently drowned on the beach near her village had.

Relieved by this simple and quick solution, she started implementing her suicide plan. She moved forward toward the exit to be the first in line to leave the train.

At the station she left the train, stepped onto the platform, and blended among the many other passengers leaving and boarding the train. Randomly, she asked someone in the crowd for directions to the sea. A man pointed the direction with his hand.

Cabiria set off on the route the man had indicated, physically feeling that the sea was not far away and that she was running in the right direction.

A strong sea breeze caressed her hair and dress. Crying hysterically, alone in the dark park and engrossed in her dark world of despair, she sprinted towards the sea—the place she had determined was going to stop her life's agony.

Suddenly, the presence of another life interrupted her focus and attention. A young couple was slowly crossing her path. Romantically embraced, the young man played a guitar while they both sang along with a popular song, both unaware of her presence, let alone her monumental problems.

Cabiria froze, composed her sobbing cries and waited for the couple to cross and clear her path. As she waited, she caught herself catching a glimpse into the lives of the couple, the young dreamers. Idealistic and in love, the couple filled the night around them with dreams, happiness, music, and song.

A broad smile appeared and stayed on Cabiria's face, accompanied by uncontrollable, running tears. Suddenly, a revelation descended upon her!

Regardless of what happened to her—*life was going on as if nothing happened!*

There would be many more other dreamers to fill her voided place. Dreamers with the same dreams, hopes, inspirations, challenges, disappointments and betrayals as hers.

Cabiria smiled and giggled. Her tears stopped. She hesitated a moment. Then turned her body 180 degrees in the opposite direction. Slowly, but surely, she began walking away from the danger of the sea and toward an opportunity, a mysterious strange town—her new life.

◻ ◻ ◻

THE MORAL OF THE STORY

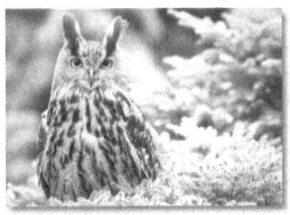

Question: What is life? Answer: Life is a dream. If there is no dream, there is no desire to live. People always dream: they want to fall in love, to meet a prince or a princess, get married, have children, buy a house, get an education, became successful at their jobs, have money, put children through college, save for retirement, and travel the world.

Try to complain to the French about your life problems and a typical answer is: "C'est la Vie." That is life. Life[1] is pain, danger, happiness, disappointment, dreams, suffering, betrayal, triumphs, opportunities, illnesses, challenges, birth, and death.

Regardless of what has happened to you, life will go on as if nothing happened. Many other people with the same dreams, disappointments and expectations as yours will fill your void. Please remember that your presence on this earth is short and temporary. And the length of your life in relation to the earth's life is just a short glitch that lasted, as a fallen star, a fraction of 1 second.

---

[1] There is also a classic book called "The Life" written by famous French writer Maupassant. Where a young woman lost her virginity.

SHORT STORY #2

WHAT IS QUALITY OF LIFE? OR, A CONVERSATION BETWEEN AN EAGLE AND A SNAKE

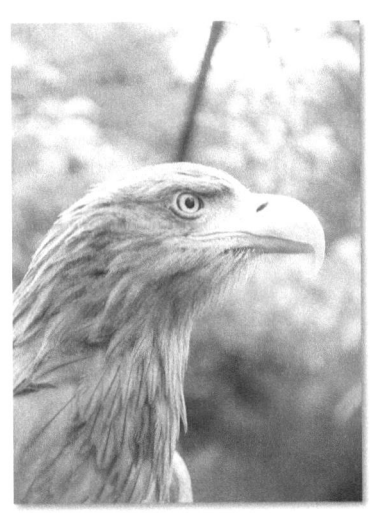
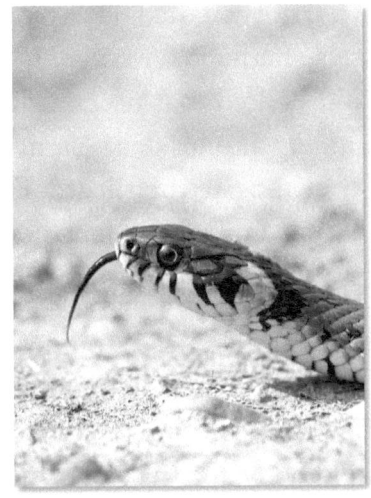

□ □ □

When I was a 4th grader attending elementary school, one of the subjects in our class curriculum was the Russian language. This subject had 2 books: a grammar book and a language book. The content of the language book had 30–40 short stories to teach young children about morality, wisdom, logic, and common sense.

An analogy of those stories was based on ancient Greek mythology, which taught people wisdom by using conversations between gods or animals. One story in my language book was designed to teach Russian children about the quality of life. The name of the story was, "A Conversation Between an Eagle and a Snake."

The story started in typical fashion…It was a hot summer afternoon. A snake, lying deep in his hole, was alert and noticed that no outside sounds from the forest were coming into his den. Alarmed and curious, he crawled out to investigate the silence. He immediately saw why—the hot sun and encroaching heat.

All the animals and his predators were paralyzed by the heat and had dispersed from his area hiding somewhere either in their dens, or holes, under leaves, or on tree branches. Feeling secure and in need of some sunning to warm up his cold body, the snake took advantage of the situation.

WHAT IS LIFE? WHAT IS HAPPINESS?

He slithered the rest of his body out from his deep hole, stretched his tail, and started enjoying the sun. Just in case one of his predators was hiding nearby, he began scanning the surrounding areas to make sure that nothing would interrupt his enjoyment.

Not far from him he saw an eagle that was hiding underneath the big branches, cooling herself from the heat. Here the snake saw an opportunity to start a conversation.

"Eagle, I feel very sorry for you," he proclaimed.

"What is there to be sorry for me about?" the eagle lazily replied.

"Well," the snake began, "I can live 300 years. But you only can live 80 years."

"Well, well...but I would not exchange even 1 day of my life for your long life of 300 years," the eagle answered.

"How come? You must be joking?" he questioned her.

"Look at you," the eagle launched into her lecture. "You are semi-blind, you cannot hear very well. You are scared of everybody and everything. The first noise you hear, you put your body into survival mode and force a rush of adrenaline.

"With the speed of light, you deposit your body back into your deep, dark hole, where for many hours you tremble in fear with your heart racing, hoping that no predators are going to fish you out from your den and eat you. To survive, you need to hunt; that is the only time when you venture outside.

"At the same time, you keep yourself alert and in fear you'll be discovered by other animals. Because of that, you never venture far away and keep a close distance to your den.

"Now, look at me. I am an eagle. I am big, strong, and majestic. I have no fears and have no predators. I am free to fly anywhere I want. Even men envy me and designed a replica of me, called an airplane. Everyday I see life and the pulse of life. I see animals, towns, people, children, and cars. I see sunrises and sunsets, forests, trees, oceans, and rivers. I live throughout changing seasons: spring and summer, autumn and winter.

"I am afraid of no one and fear nothing. That is why I would not exchange even 1 day of my life for 300 years of your fearful, stationary, and empty existence in that dark deep hole."

Let's consider a few examples applicable to the above conversation between the eagle and the snake.

EXAMPLE #1

In 1980s, there was a historic exodus of population from Russian villages and small towns. A trend swept across the Soviet Union, to live in big cities where jobs, apartments, schools, and entertainment venues were all located in one place, to improve the quality of life.

The world was progressing, changing, and moving forward. These world changes brought television and the media to every Russian home. The population became informed and aware about the world around them.

They became sophisticated and wanted to be part of the world's progress. Even more, they wanted to live a high quality of life, which they could find only in big cities where jobs, opportunities, education, and entertainment were all in one place. Hundreds of thousands of Russian villages and small towns were simply abandoned.

When I learned about this exodus, my nostalgia kicked in. During my childhood years, I spent several unforgettable, magical summer vacations in some of those villages. My grandma Anna would take me with her to see her relatives and occupied herself socializing and making fruits and vegetables preserves for the winter. I was free to do whatever I wanted and spent my energy playing all day with other children, running barefoot all day, swimming in the river, and eating fruit in the orchards.

Our evenings were spent in the village center where local teenagers entertained themselves. Boys played accordions, guitars, and mandolins, and girls danced and sang. We, the younger children, learned from them how to dance and memorized and sang all their songs. I wrote those songs into an album and when I came back to school in September, I gave my "Songs Album" to my class teacher as my summer assignment.

Recently, I asked my brother Victor, who lives in Odessa on the Black Sea, to drive to those villages to see what became of them after 20–30 years of abandonment. Soon he called me with his report.

The villages were gone—only the walls of houses, made from concrete blocks, remained. The forest moved in and took over the abandoned places. The entire place was covered with vegetation, with only the cemeteries maintained by visiting relatives continuing to take care of their loved ones' graves.

In the evening, wolves were howling, cutting through the thick silence for many kilometers on end. Except for wolves, and some small animals, Victor saw no humans around.

EXAMPLE #2

How and why the population of Paris live a high quality of life?

Let's look at Paris, which is a familiar city to many Americans tourists. In Paris, a 160 sq. foot small studio (such a small studio probably does not exist in the USA) is in big demand, stays on the market for just a few hours, and usually sells for over $300,000. Why?

WHAT IS LIFE? WHAT IS HAPPINESS?

The human life is outside, not inside of that box (i.e., that apartment or house). The French live their lives as eagles outside, not as snakes inside their holes.

Why do the French live 6 years longer than Americans do? They have almost no depression, no type 2 diabetes, or arthritis, or asthma, and very few of the French finish their lives in nursing homes. They worship the sun, air, and strolls in the city.

Plus, French and all Europeans take their high quality of life for granted, including services like free health care, free education, cheap housing, pensions, retirement at age 60–62, a 35-hour workweek, and 1-month paid vacations. Unfortunately, the USA does not have these important elements to provide a high quality of life for its citizens.

Why are the French so skinny, even after they eat the same junk food as Americans? This is very often a topic on American TV. The answer is a very simple one. The French spend their time outside of their homes—on streets, in cafes, bars, or just strolling the streets talking to friends, complaining, learning from each other, and solving each other's problems. They come home late at night just to sleep.

A lazy stroll for 1 hour a day takes energy from the body, approximately 150 calories. That is a weight loss =1.5 lbs/month, or 18 pounds per year.[1] No dieting, no taking any diet pills. In short, the French are losing 18 pounds per year just by enjoying their lives and being outside, not inside.

And how much happiness do the French get by seeing the pulse of everyday life—people, children, animals, streets, buildings, trees, flowers, and bushes when they are walking, sitting in cafes, talking with friends and strangers, solving each other's problems, and dreaming? Seeing how the weather and seasons are changing. It is priceless.

THE MORAL OF THE STORY

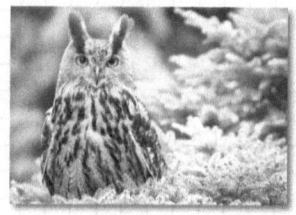

"A Conversation Between an Eagle and a Snake. Or, What is the Quality of Life?" An eagle lives a high quality of life; she lives and flies outside and sees the world and life around her. She sees cities, towns, people, children, animals, cars, buildings, trees, bushes, rivers, and oceans. She sees sunrises and sunsets, how spring changes to summer, then fall, then winter.

The snake lives a poor quality of life; he spends all his life in a dark, deep den from where he ventures outside only to hunt for his food.

WHAT IS LIFE? WHAT IS HAPPINESS?

Question: how do you want to live your life? Outside or inside? Who would you like to be: an eagle and live 80 years, or a snake and live 300 years?

The above wise stories teach us that a high quality of life is outside where the eagle flies and lives, and not inside where the snake spends his life lying all day in his deep and dark den.

Why do you think you are always dreaming about European vacations or about a faraway place being on some tropical island under the sun, surrounded by exotic flora and fauna? How many times have you pretended to be one of your favorite heroes from books you read or movies you saw?

You, like your heroes, could be walking wide boulevards among the crowd in some far away metropolitan city, consumed by the city's life, passing buildings, cafes, shop windows, wrapped up in noises coming from city transportation and crowds.

You see the everyday life: people, children, animals, cars, buildings, lights, trees, and flowers. You could be enjoying the weather: warm, cold, rain, or snow. Notice what season it is now...Summer, fall, winter, or spring?

And dream, dream, dream...In your dreams you can be anyone or anything. You have the same spirit and desires as an eagle does. That is why you try to create some rare moments to enjoy a high quality of life and be a participant in this magical life on this earth.

In short, life is outside, not inside. Where should a person live? The answer is very simple. Live in a big compact metropolitan city; rent an apartment there. Walk or use public transportation to get to work, school, home, entertainment, and shopping. Walk the streets just to see the rhythm of life. Enjoy the weather. Notice season changes. And dream, dream, dream...

Do not go home directly from work; instead, take a walk or detour for 4–5 blocks, walk with the crowd or sit on a bench. Do as Europeans do every day, especially the French who are familiar to the majority of Americans. They live in big cities, in small apartments where they go back home late at night only to sleep.

---

[1] Where: (150 calories spend on walking 1 hour x 30 days) ÷ 3,000 calories/pound =1.5 lbs/month. Or, 18 lbs weight loss per year = (1.5 lbs/month x 12 month).

SHORT STORY

#3

A FOOL AND A COMMON SENSE. OR, 5 DONUTS AND 1 BAGEL

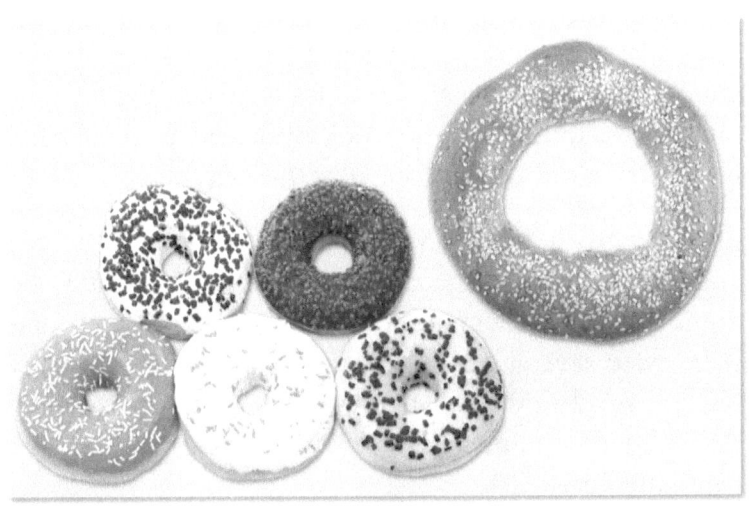

□ □ □

This wise riddle was one of the stories in my elementary school Russian language class. It begins like this...

After Sunday service was over, churchgoers hurried outside and dispersed in all directions. Not Ivan. The farmer and a chubby man in his early 30s did some thinking. What activity should he pursue next and what should he do for the rest of his Sunday? He couldn't come up with anything, but that did not discourage him.

Today he was free; he had no obligations to fulfill and no farm work to tend to. Time was at his disposal. Lazily, he began walking down the street towards the town center, and kicking some small stones lying on the sidewalk along the way.

After a few blocks, to his left side he noticed some activity going on. People from all directions were heading towards one big building. Curiosity took over, and Ivan changed his direction towards the center of this activity.

Once he reached the area, he mixed with other people and became one of the crowd. Following the others, he found himself in the middle of the farmers market. Around there were several long rows, each populated with many big and small wooden stands where local farmers proudly displayed their numerous crops of different varieties of fruits and vegetables.

WHAT IS LIFE? WHAT IS HAPPINESS?

Soon the smell of grilled pork together with cinnamon and vanilla from freshly baked goods reached his nostrils. It awakened his appetite; he felt hungry and decided it was time to have lunch.

Following the smell of the food, he came across a pavilion designated just for that purpose, fresh cooked food. Entering the pavilion, he took off his hat and prepared to have lunch there. He picked up a menu. Just for a starter, he decided to have his favorite—freshly baked crispy bread with melted butter on top.

Before he finished his bread, the smell of hardy beef soup started teasing his appetite. He bought that, together with some rice, as a side dish and ate immediately, but his hunger did not subside. Next, he bought and ate 5 donuts, washing them down with 2 glasses of milk.

Still the hunger was there. His stomach craved more food, but at the same time he felt tired from digesting so much food. "Now, let me try 1 bagel with cream cheese!" he said loudly and picked up his list of options. After he finished the bagel, he suddenly felt 100% full. His hunger was gone completely.

Amazed, he sat on the bench, but then kicked himself hard on the head as the realization set in. "What a fool I am! I ate huge amounts of food and wasted a lot of my money on it when buying just 1 single bagel with cheese could have completely satisfied my hunger!" he proclaimed in disappointment.

Ivan, being a farmer, typically worked all day from dawn to dusk on his farm doing physical tasks associated with looking after his cattle and his fields. This physical job required a lot of energy. And from where did he get his energy to perform such enormous tasks? From food. He needed to consume much more food than, for example, a man who works in an office sitting all day in his chair.

Ivan did manual farm work all day and had no time to pursue additional education, or read many books. That is why his brain did not have enough information to analyze unfamiliar problems and find a correct and simple answer to them.

Sometimes I watched *the Court TV* to witness how many middle-aged people do not have common sense, or logic.

EXAMPLE #1
A woman hit a car that was behind a van. If she looked, she could see it. But she had the "right of way" and kept driving. Now she is in a courtroom asking the judge to order the driver, whose car she hit, to pay for her car repair.

The judge told her that it was her fault, not the man's whose car she hit. She was not convinced and kept repeating, even after the verdict, that it was not her fault and that she had the "right of way."

EXAMPLE #2
A middle-aged woman, the plaintiff, hit another car and damaged both cars, her own car and the other vehicle.

Then, she filed a lawsuit asking the other car's driver, the defendant who was a middle-aged man, to pay for her car repairs.

The defendant, who had no driver's license, filed a countersuit asking the plaintiff to pay for his car damages. The judge ruled for the defendant, and against the plaintiff. The plaintiff could not believe that the judge had ruled against her.

After the verdict, she and her husband still blamed the defendant; she insisted it was not her fault. In unison, they kept reiterating: "He (the defendant) has no driver's license and has no business being on the road."

□ □ □

THE MORAL OF THE STORY

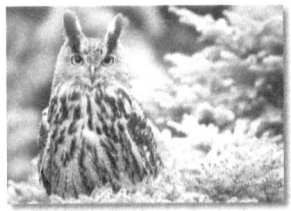

A person should have a major skill. It's called common sense, or logic. To solve every problem, whether big, small, personal, business, national, or local, requires this major skill. Common sense or logic could be retrieved from a person's brain folder, provided that a person has enough information, knowledge, and experience stored in his brain database.

That is why children cannot solve adult problems; they have not lived long enough to accumulate a sufficient volume of information in their brain folder to help them find solutions to adult problems. That is how and why people become wiser as they grow older. By the time they are seniors, some will be wise enough to solve even the most difficult of life's problems.

Examples of this are Nobel Prize winners. These are people with extremely high intelligence, who, if they live long enough, may became Nobel Laureates in their 70s and 80s. By that time, their brain database has accumulated enough of the information and knowledge needed to solve significant national or world problems.

SHORT STORY #4

THERE IS NO ROYAL ROAD TO KNOWLEDGE. OR, A LESSON FROM ALEXANDER THE GREAT

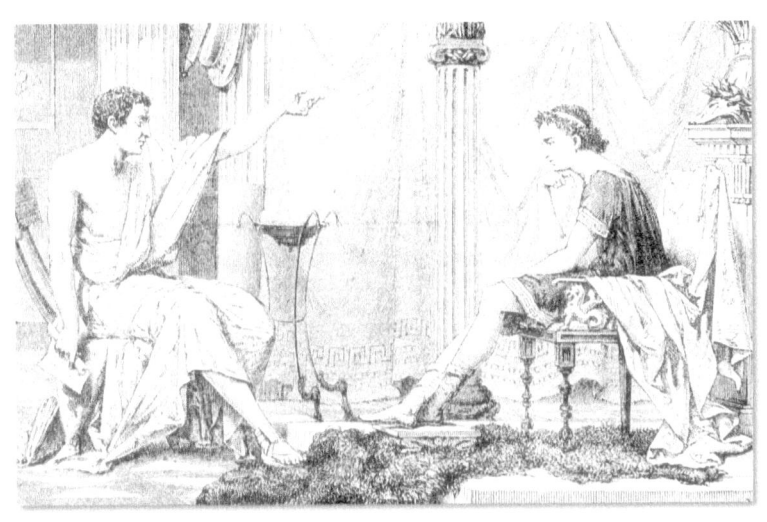

☐ ☐ ☐

When my class started taking algebra in the 5th grade, our teacher reassured us that algebra was a simple subject. "Algebra is just an extension of arithmetic," she told us. She reminded us that in arithmetic, we dealt with numbers whereas in algebra there were formulas, theorems, axioms, and symbols to replace the numbers and all of them required memorization.[1]

If you do not remember a correct formula, theorem, or axiom, you cannot solve the problem correctly, and the result will be wrong.

For 1 week, we children memorized theorems and axioms, and then applied them to our assigned homework problems. The following week, our teacher discovered that the results in our homework were alarming, as the majority of us had written the wrong answers.

When she asked each of us to recite the theorems and axioms we were supposed to have correctly memorized, very few of us gave her a correct answer.

To solve both, her and our problems, our teacher told us a story citing the laws of life: responsibility and hard work. She said we children were growing up, while at the same time our responsibilities were increasing and also our need to work hard in life.

The difficult subjects had only just started. Algebra was the most important subject that required responsibility, effort, energy, memorization, repetition, and time.

She warned that if we did not memorize all formulas, theorems, and axioms correctly, then we could not solve problems correctly, and the result would be predictable. We would fail algebra and would have to repeat the 5th grade.

To emphasize her point, she told us a story about Alexander the Great. She explained how, a young prince, Alexander, or Alexander the Great as he is popularly known, learned his algebra and math subjects.

Alexander's father, Philip, was a great King of Macedonia. His father brought the best teachers and tutors in the kingdom to his palace to teach and tutor the young Alexander in many different subjects. One of his teachers was Aristotle, who taught the young prince several subjects, including math and science.

Every day, Aristotle gave Alexander an assignment to solve problems and memorize formulas, theorems, and axioms. In the beginning, Alexander was respectful and was learning fast. Soon, he recognized that homework took up all of his time, energy, and effort and left no time to play.

Alexander started looking for a way out of having to learn such difficult subjects.

During his next math lesson, Alexander threw his books into the air and declared, "I am a future king! I do not need to study so hard all the time as commoners; let them study, not I!" Aristotle answered him in one sentence, "There is no royal road to knowledge."

This means that knowledge does not discriminate. Regardless of who you are—be it a king, or a commoner—to learn something requires a lot of effort, energy, repetition, memorization, and focus.

Alexander understood Aristotle's law of life and started studying seriously and hard. In the end, he developed a great desire for knowledge, was an avid reader, and loved philosophy, science and art, and debates. But Alexander had a little interest in sports and games. He became a king at age 20.

Alexander the Great died at the age of 32. Yet, during his short life (356 BC–323 BC), he never lost a battle and is considered to be the greatest military genius of all time.

His genius and his undefeated victories came from the extensive tutoring he received from the best minds in the kingdom in science, math, philosophy, medicine, and logic.

His broad and hard learning produced his great logic, knowledge, and common sense and won him all his battles. He believed in himself and in his own destiny.

THE MORAL OF THE STORY

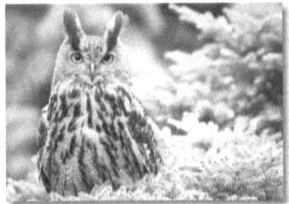

There is no royal road to knowledge. Knowledge does not discriminate. A king or a commoner can have access to knowledge through constant learning when they apply hard work, effort, and focus.

To reinforce the above statement, let's take an example of learning a foreign language, say French. Let's take 2 individuals: one is a prince; another, a typical average person. Let's say they both started learning French at the same time.

After 6–12 months, let's see who knows French better—a prince or a commoner? It is very easy to find out. As soon as they start speaking, you would be able to hear who knew French better.

Only the person who puts in persistent time, energy, and effort and memorizes French all day and everyday could speak better. The status of "prince" or "governor" or "president" or "PhD" will not help and has no relevance to the ability to speak French well. Nor does luck or opportunity help.

Working hard and employing memorization and repetition every day for weeks and months—is the effort required to do the job.

---

[1] Arithmetic deals with particular numbers, for example:
$(20 + 4)^2 = 20^2 + 2 \times 20 \times 4 + 4^2 = 576$.
Algebra has formulas and symbols. The formula remains true no matter what particular number may replace the symbols a and b.
Lets convert the above arithmetic into algebra formula and symbols:
$(a + b)^2 = a^2 + 2 \times a \times b + b^2$.

SHORT STORY

#5

EVERYONE HAS THE SAME AMOUNT OF ENERGY; IT ALL DEPENDS WHERE YOU PUT OR CHANNEL IT

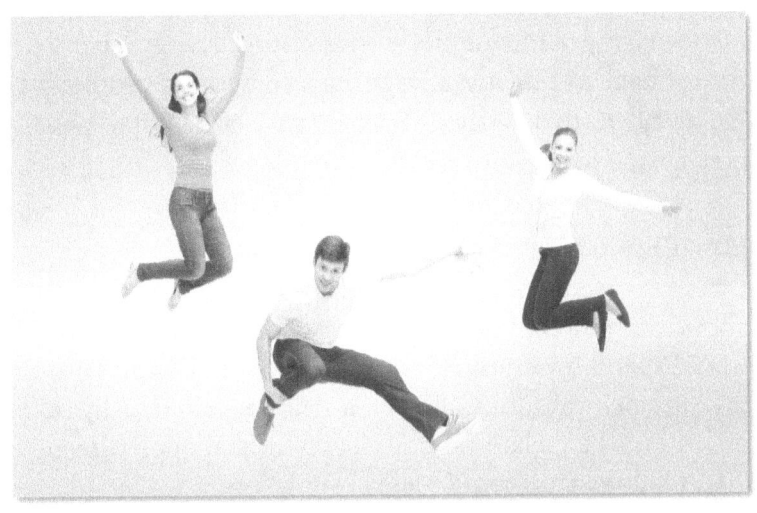

MY GRANDPA'S CONCERN

This was the year I became a teenager, and my summer vacations were quickly approaching. This event brought huge concern and uneasiness to my grandpa Vasily. He reached for his cigarettes more often, started thinking longer, and took several trips across the city to visit some of our relatives that he had not seen in years.

Something was bothering him, and he was determined to find a solution to this problem. His concern was that as a teenager, I would start doing teenage things: smoking, drinking, attending 24-hour beach parties, running after boys, and get bored from doing nothing.

Grandpa's problem was, I soon learned, where to channel his teenage granddaughter's combusting energy? He was determined to put my energy into something productive. He decided that I should learn new skills that would prepare me for my life and adulthood.

MY YOUNGER YEARS

Before my teen years, my grandpa never seemed concerned about the amount of energy I had or where and how I would spend my summer vacations. It was typical. During my summer vacations, grandma Anna would usually take me to visit her relatives in a village located approximately 80–90 kilometers from Odessa.

There she spent time socializing and making preserves of fruits and vegetables for the winter. As for me, I was free to run barefoot with my village friends, exploring the life and world around us.

We basked in the warm water in the river until the crawfish pinched our bodies. In pain and fear, we would run to the banks of the river screaming and looking for adults to help us to unlock the crawfish hanging from our bodies. Still in pain and agony, we switched our activities to other adventures. We scaled orchard trees for peaches, cherries, pears, and apples that we ate right there and then.

In the evenings, still bubbling with energy, sometimes we did bad things. We descended upon a watermelon farm to steal watermelons and teased the guard. He was prepared for us. Armed with a long shotgun loaded with coarse salt, he would fire at us, aiming at the lower parts of our bodies.

Yelling and screaming from pain, we would run toward the river where we would sit in the water until the salt particles dissolved in our wounds and the pain diminished. Then 1 week later, we would forget about this scary adventure and do it again.

And the movies were magic! Once a week, a big truck with movie equipment would arrive in the village entertainment center to show a movie on a big screen. Many villagers would come to see the movies, along with all the older children.

We young children did not buy tickets; instead we sneaked among the adults for free. Instinctively, we understood that as long as we did not occupy seats reserved for people with tickets, we could watch movies sitting on the pathway stairs and windows.

We did, and after the presentation was over, we exited, happy and animated as we continued discussing and imitating our movie heroes for the rest of the evening and the following days.

The majority of our evenings were spent in the yard of the village City Hall. There, almost every evening, local teenagers would gather accompanied by accordions, harmonicas, and drums; they would dance and sing.

We young children observed and listened to what the teens were doing and copied them. We memorized and sang their popular songs to ourselves, and we learned how to dance from them.

I wrote every one of their songs into my "Song Album" and also collected flora and fauna for another album. In September, when I went back to school, I turned both albums in as my summer's homework assignment.

Nothing lasts forever, not even my happy childhood. Every summer I grew older, distancing myself from my childhood years and headed towards my teens.

TEENAGE ENERGY

When I became a teenager, my attitude dramatically changed. I no longer had any interest in traveling with my grandma to the village for my summer vacations. Now my world revolved around my city friends.

Here is where my grandpa interfered, putting the brakes on my teen activities. His law of life was that, "Everyone has approximately the same amount of energy; it all depends where you put or channel it." He put this law into practice and applied it to me.

One evening, grandpa put on his best suit and his velour hat, which he reserved for special occasions, and asked me to go with him to the home of one of our relatives, Vladimir, a chief financial officer at a local factory.

That evening grandpa told Vladimir that I was a "straight A" student, an honor student, and had been since 1st grade. To reinforce his point, grandpa showed Vladimir all the achievements and awards that I had received to date. I was embarrassed, but grandpa was successful in his plan—I got a summer job in Vladimir's factory.

CHANNELING MY ENERGY INTO MY SUMMER JOBS

Vladimir tried me out in all of his departments: financial, accounts receivable and payable, and strategic planning to help his staff. To all the other employees, I was just a child, or like their daughter.

They liked me and treated me well, but gave me plenty of different work most of which they did not like to do, or was too monotonous or needed to be done quickly.

I was a very shy child, respectful of adults, a hard worker, and fearful of making errors. What employers did not know was that with every new task they gave me to complete, I would go into panic mode.

Some of their words I did not understand when hearing them for the first time, let alone being able to complete their assignments.

For example: workers' outputs, accounts receivable, balance payable, productivity, and workers turnover. I was 13 years old and my brain had a very small storage of information to help me.

I would get scared and panic with each new assignment I received and start to worry. How could I complete it? What would my employers think of me if I could not deliver the assignment to them? How could I erase all those scary thoughts from my mind and stop worrying?

To raise my self-esteem, I turned to my childhood heroes: Tom Sawyer and Huckleberry Finn. What would they do in my place? I was sure that they would not be panicked.

Instead, they would attack the problem head on. So from then on, I pretended I was Tom or Huckleberry. When scary thoughts came to my mind, I commanded that they leave. When I was unsure of myself, I would tell my brain: *Stop it, and stop disseminating your energy on worries; instead, put all your energy and attention into this one and only focal point—the assignment in front of you.* It worked.

More summers followed, and over the next few years, I learned to be creative, to focus, and to be enthusiastic. In addition, I learned some other skills: accounting, finance, and strategic planning. All those skills were added to my brain storage. Now, I was far ahead of my friends and later, my peers.

Thanks to the wisdom of my grandpa Vasily, those skills later enhanced my career, my life, and changed my destiny.

During my teenage years, my grandpa Vasily was secretly implementing his long-held personal dream and his legacy. That I, his granddaughter, would became self-sufficient and would not have to depend on a husband for support.

To achieve that, he wanted me to become a structural engineer and design buildings, bridges, and subways and by doing so, leave monuments after myself. He was my mentor, supporter, and my biggest fan.

When attending civil engineering school (my university was located just 4 blocks from my grandparents' apartment), I was living with my grandparents and my grandpa was actively involved in my studies and that of my friends.

THE MORAL OF THE STORY

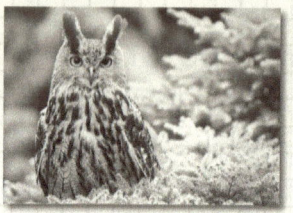

My grandpa Vasily's one law of life was: "Everyone has approximately the same amount of energy, it all depends where you put or channel it."

In my case, I owe many thanks to my grandpa Vasily's wisdom; he channeled my combustive teenage energy into a productive outlet—summer jobs. There, I learned new skills that later helped me to solve many of my adult problems, thus changing my life and my destiny. From that point, I learned to love to work and could not live without working; work was life and I wanted to be an active participant in it.

Lesson in point for today's children, teenagers, and young adults: During their critical development in their young and teen years, they are learning no new skills. Instead, their brains and their storage database are "doped" due to Facebook, Twitter,

Instagram, texting, apps, hip-hop, Disney World, fantasies, *Dancing with the Stars*, video games, e-mails.

Once they became adults, their brains will be empty. Their brains will have no information on how to live, survive, find a job, work, invent, behave, or run their homes, let alone run their country. They need to have their energy channeled into productive pursuits that will ultimately benefit them down the road in their lives.

SHORT STORY

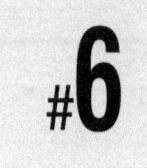

OUR MIND IS A TAPE RECORDER

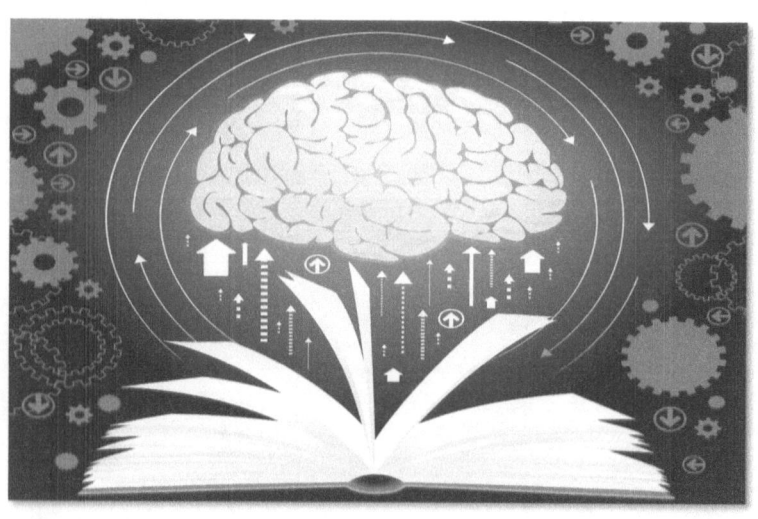

WHAT IS LIFE? WHAT IS HAPPINESS?

◻ ◻ ◻

"Our mind is a tape recorder!" That is how my professor in the "Strength of Materials" class started his lecture one day. This proclamation deviated from the usual course subject, and we students were puzzled.

His usual way was running from one blackboard to another, populating the surfaces with intricate formulas. Then he would stop for a moment and scan the amphitheatre where over 400 civil engineering students were scattered, taking note of whether we were quick and bright enough to write down his formulas and solutions in our notebooks.

Behind his back we called him "I-beam" and "Mephistopheles." The I-beam was his innovation trap to fail students; designing an I-beam was the pre-requisite before taking his exam. We called him "Mephistopheles" because that is how he looked to us.

He had grey piercing eyes with heavy eyebrows; he wore a black turtleneck sweater with black pants and bounced his tall and skinny frame between 3 blackboards, intimidating us. He also had a notebook filled with notes on every student.

Because of his presence, the environment in the amphitheatre was always stressful and tense. Angst was the prevailing mood, at least when students were not altogether scared to death of him. Who wouldn't be?

He could destroy the lives of hundreds of students by failing them. The fate of many in our class, we knew from previous statistics, would be the same. That is, many students would fail his subject, and thus not graduate.

There was very little anyone could do about it though because this professor was a prominent scientist who had made a huge contribution in his field. For his contribution, he had been rewarded as a tenured professor for life. Consequently, it was as if he now was a supreme power in the university—power he did not hesitate to invoke.

On this day, he deviated from his subject when addressing his wary audience with a simple question: "Has anyone noticed this recent trend, whereby people use tape recorders to learn foreign languages while they are asleep?"

He paused, waiting for someone to answer. Fearful, no one volunteered an answer, lest they put themselves before this one-man firing squad, or attract attention. He looked up at the students seated in the gallery; they too were silent.

He knew all too well that the gallery was overcrowded with students who were not sure whether they would pass his subject and, therefore, kept their distance as a result. Students were suspicious and went on high alert.

"He is up to no good," I thought. My survival instincts stirred, my body tensed, and my mind focused with laser-like precision on his presentation. That is why I remember his "Our mind is a tape recorder" speech vividly, as if it was yesterday.

The professor continued addressing the nervous amphitheatre. "You see," he stated, "this discovery was made just recently in England. A maid, who had worked for a prominent English family, fell into a stair shaft and badly injured her head. She was rushed by ambulance to a hospital in one of London's slums. She was given emergency medical care but was not expected to survive. She was near-comatose, ran a high fever, and talked in her sleep.

"The hospital staff noticed that she talked in a language they had never heard before. She was also reciting poetry in this strange tongue. Their curiosity was overwhelming, so they invited a linguistics professor to try and unlock the mystery. He did. The maid was reciting poems in a very old version of English—a Saxony version of English which only a limited number of people know today.

"Now hospital staff thought she could be a very important person with a noble background versus being a mere maid. Shortly thereafter, they transferred her to one of the best hospitals in London, redoubling their efforts to save her. Meanwhile, a tape recorder continued to record everything she said.

"When she recovered, the first question the staff asked her was "Who are you? And how did you learn Saxon English?" The answer was that she had no idea what they were talking about. She did not even know that such a language existed, let alone know she could speak it and recite poems in it.

"In the end, the mystery was solved. How? Many years ago, this maid was working for one professor who was a specialist in linguistics—in Saxon English. While working all day in his library, he would read loudly, even sometimes reciting poems in Saxon.

"As she was serving him meals at breakfast and lunch while cleaning and bringing him his tea or lingering in his library completing her chores, this professor would read and recite Saxon English loudly.

"Subconsciously, without her knowledge or input, her mind, like a tape recorder, kept recording this professor's words. Then, after she finished her day job in his home, she would go back to her own home where on top of the Saxon English language she heard in the professor's house, her mind would record new information and bury the Saxon English learning in another area of her brain.

"For the rest of her life, she probably would never have known that somewhere deep in her brain she stored these Saxon poems and language.

"Of course, all that changed when she fell into that stair shaft, cracking her head and injuring her brain in the area where this Saxon language had been stored subconsciously.

Now, it was exposed and rose to the surface and poured out in her subconscious talk.

"Hence, a discovery had been made—our mind is a tape recorder. It constantly records everything it hears around us. By the time a person is an adult, their brain has already accumulated scores of information from tape recordings.

"Old information is buried while new information is recorded on top of or over this old information. To retrieve particular old information buried deep in the storage of our brains, one needs to pinpoint precisely in our brain where that information is located.

"In the case of this English maid, her brain was cracked (from the fall) in the area where the Saxon language was stored. Now, this language was easily accessible without any effort, which was how this maid, in her unconscious state, was able to recite the Saxon poems and language."

To emphasize this point, our professor of "Strength of Materials" gave us another logical analogy, explaining why young children, when learning a foreign language, can learn it virtually effortlessly in weeks rather than months. This was because their tape recorder minds are still almost empty.

New information is located close to the surface of the mind, and for a child to retrieve it, in this case to speak a foreign language, for example French, is very easy. Then, let's take the same child who, for the next 3 years never spoke French.

The result is the child will forget French completely. This is due to the fact that for 3 years, on top of the earlier learned French language, many layers of new information have been recorded, and thus have buried the French beneath it.

My personal examples: The professor in the above theory seems to be right.

EXAMPLE #1

When we came to the USA, our eldest son spoke only Russian and Swahili. We spoke Russian at home. He learned Swahili from Hadiga, his aya or nanny,[1] who spoke only Swahili. So he learned it from her, from our housekeeper, and from other children and adults in Dar es Salaam, Tanzania. He not only spoken Swahili, he also knew Swahili jokes. But he did not know any English.

In the USA, to speed up his learning of English, we stopped speaking Russian at home. Very quickly he learned English and caught up with his classmates. But 3–4 years later he has forgotten Russian and Swahili completely; he could not remember even one word.

EXAMPLE #2

The same happened with my eldest grandson. For 3 years he went to a French-American school where all subjects were in French; he knew French and sang French songs. Then, after 3 years, he transferred to an English school. A few years later, he has forgotten French completely.

Thereafter, this professor summarized his conclusions on this topic by drawing an illustration on the blackboard of a comparison of the size of a human brain versus the size of our consciousness. The average brain weighs about 3 pounds. It is approximately 15 cm. in length.

But the area of consciousness is merely a pin point. On top of the brain the professor inserted a small dot and drew a line out of the brain to show that the size of consciousness is very small in relation to the size of our brains, which is why we have difficulty when retrieving old, deeply located information, knowledge, skills, thoughts, or memories.

□ □ □

THE MORAL OF THE STORY

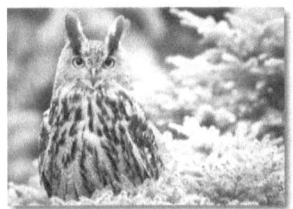

Our mind is a tape recorder. Huge stores of data are recorded in it. The storage is nearly unquantifiable and no computer designed today can imitate it, let alone replace even a small part of the intricate storage in the human mind.

The more information a person stores in his mind and brain, the more opportunity he has to solve life's problems and to survive under the most difficult and challenging circumstances.

That is how and why our brains perform these wonders. It finds solutions to all our problems, provided we populate our brain storage with important and needed information for everyday existence.

Every day, our brains are putting new information into its storage.

Question: How can the youth of today survive, let alone run the nation and economy one day when the older generation dies off?

The fact is that today, the younger generation keep their brains "doped" by talking gossips all day on iPhones and texting while engaged in trivial pursuits. They are focused 24/7 on Facebook, Twitter, YouTube, the Kardashians, America's Got Talent, Disney fantasies, video games, Skype, email, and many more not important pursuits.

The mind is a tape recorder, or a well, where intellect is stored along with information, skills, and

WHAT IS LIFE? WHAT IS HAPPINESS?

knowledge. Without intellect, a person is empty, ignorant, and unsophisticated, and when intellect dies, the nation dies.

---

[1] Nanny, or Aya is a name for nanny in East Africa. Nannies look after a child permanently for longer hours, regardless of the presence of the parents.

SHORT STORY #7

WHAT IS HAPPINESS? OR, WHAT WERE THE HAPPIEST YEARS OF YOUR LIFE?

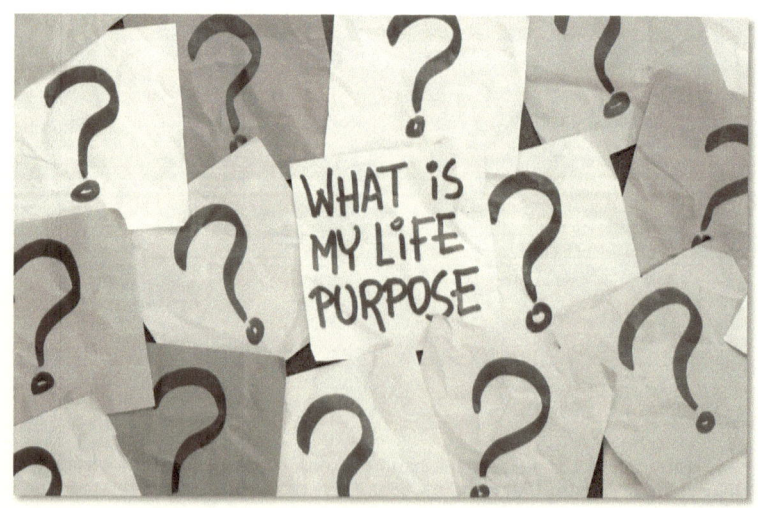

WHAT IS LIFE? WHAT IS HAPPINESS?

□ □ □

One evening, my eldest son suddenly asked me: "Mom, what were the happiest years of your life?" I did not hesitate—I knew the answer. "When we were living in Africa," I said.

My answer stunned him. His eyes started beaming. A rush of emotion sprinted him to his feet, he started pacing the living room, looking at me in disbelief. "Something is wrong with you! In Africa we were poor!" he declared.

That evening, I went to bed earlier than usual and retrieved a segment of my life when we were living in Africa.

THE MOST EXCITING YEARS OF MY GENERATION
The 1950s–1980s were the most technologically advanced years in human civilization in the 20th century. Historic, advanced, exciting, awesome, passionate, and turbulent years of my generation.

There was a Cold War. The 2 superpowers, the USA and the Soviet Union, were in fierce competition for technological progress and dominance of the world. Who was going to win: capitalism or socialism? My generation was very lucky: we lived during some great historic events, technological breakthroughs, and exciting times.

In the summer of 1957, rock 'n' roll had come onto the scene, as Elvis Presley's hit records "Don't be Cruel" and

"Hound Dog" swept across the world and captured the young imaginations.

On October 4, 1957, the Soviet Union launched Sputnik, the world's 1st satellite. It orbited the earth and transmitted signals across the world. Sputnik (Companion in English) emitted *"Beep...Beep...Beep"* signals back to earth, they were heard around the world.

The world was shocked; it did not expect such technological progress for many generations. Sputnik circled the globe and triggered the development of space programs and arms race.

On April 12, 1961, Russian cosmonaut Yuri Gagarin was the first man in space. In his spacecraft Vostok-1, he traveled to space and orbited the earth.

He became a legend of this historical progress for the whole world. Even today, over 50 years later, the majority of people on this planet know who Yuri Gagarin was.

Space programs and arms races produced the greatest inventions and innovations in human history, and thousands of them spilled into civilian industries. Long distance telecommunications, artificial intelligence, robotics, digital cameras, LED chips, microwave ovens, insulin pumps, cardiac pacemakers, smoke detectors, water filters, and thousands of other technological advances mushroomed and improved the quality of life for every person.

WHAT IS LIFE? WHAT IS HAPPINESS?

The whole world was in bloom from these new inventions.

There was also the Olympics that produced fierce sports competition between the 2 superpowers and their satellites. It became a competition between capitalism and socialism. Life, dreams, and excitement radiated throughout all 6 continents.

Dreams were in the air. Technological development seemed like it had no limits. Soon, we were sure, we would all fly on spacecrafts to the moon for our vacations. I was in love with this life and was an active participant in this life excitement.

The African continent was rapidly changing. It threw off the chains of colonial powers, and one by one African countries became free, independent, and in charge of their own destinies. This historic event attracted many Western and Eastern specialists and intellectuals to Africa.

Hundreds of thousands of engineers, architects, teachers, economists, physicians, technicians, and Peace Corp volunteers came to Africa to help build their superstructures, economy, education, health care, and independence.

At that time, I graduated from the Odessa Civil Engineering University, Odessa, in the Soviet Union, and my then husband, Chrys, received his medical degree from the Odessa Medical University. And with our 10-month-old son, we embarked on our journey to Africa.

RWANDA, CENTRAL AFRICA

We arrived in Kigali, the capital city of Rwanda, Central Africa in September 1967. Rwanda was a former Belgian colony, a French-speaking country, and one of the most scenic and bucolic countries in Africa.

It was called Africa's Switzerland and "Land of a thousand hills." The longest river in the world, the Nile, originates in Rwanda, and its jungles are the home of Mountain Gorillas (Kwita Izina). Rwanda is also the most densely populated country in Africa, and the native country of my then husband, Chrysologue, or Chrys for short.

Young, naive, inexperienced, and vulnerable, I arrived with only one idealistic intention—to help Rwanda design and build national wealth: buildings, hotels, factories, roads and bridges, so that years later, before I died, I would be able to look back on my life and be proud that I did not live a selfish life. Instead, I made some contribution to other people; in this case, to this African nation.

Little did I know that fate had different plans in her store for me and was waiting to ambush me with monumental challenges and life-threatening events.

It all started badly from our very first day in Kigali. After that, everything just went downhill. The Ministry of Labor refused to give me a job. "We've never had a woman civil engineer here before and do not need one now," the administrator told me bluntly. As I was leaving the ministry, panic set in. How were we going to live and survive without jobs? The answer was a simple one.

I must find a job. On the next block, I did. Tall cranes, like the heads of giraffes, were popping out across the city, signaling that building construction in Kigali was booming.

I stopped at several construction sites and from their billboards wrote down names of some engineering design companies. Then I asked a few construction managers to give me names of the large and popular companies in Kigali. They referred me to one Belgian-Italian engineering company.

Following their suggestions, I walked into the company, introduced myself, and simply asked if they had a job for me. They were very receptive and explained that they had a great need for structural engineers, whom they usually imported from Europe and paid all relocation expenses for them, including their families. And here I was, already in Kigali, with no time wasted and without any expense to the company.

They were glad to hire me. They unrolled on the drawing board a hotel's field drawings, and assigned it to me on the spot. They explained that I was going to design this multi-story hotel in Kigali, called L'Ambassadeur ("Hotel Ambassador" in English). That was my project. The rest of the afternoon, a chief engineer and an architect gave me some important data for my design.

What a day it was! Clouds of fear engulfed my body. For several hours, I was bombarded by French language I was unaccustomed to, with many technical words I was hearing for the first time, but made an effort to guess what they meant. Overwhelmed and exhausted, my mind ran and survived on adrenaline.

In the end, 5 p.m. arrived and I was free to go to our temporary home where one family, upon our arrival, took us to stay with them. Outside, I felt dizzy and nauseous. I detoured to a construction site, where I threw up. But, I had no time to fall apart and had no other alternative. The next morning, stoically, like a soldier, I marched back to my new job.

With every passing day, my situation at work became easier, my adjustment to hearing all day French eased. Soon my difficulties disappeared—I became used to the environment and loved my work.

My salary was big, and was paid in US dollars, not in Rwandese franks (later, because I had dollars, we were able to escape Rwanda). We received a new, furnished and free of charge 2-bedroom apartment.

As for Chrys, his job prospects were not so good. He was a physician and Rwanda had socialized medicine, free to all citizens. All physicians worked for the government and were assigned to places where there was a need for them,

WHAT IS LIFE? WHAT IS HAPPINESS?

not where physicians particularly wanted to work. Plus, Chrys was a Tutsi.

In power now were the Hutu. The Hutu were paranoid that the Tutsi were going to seize power from them at any moment. They had reason to be alarmed. Before Belgium colonized Rwanda after World War I (WWI, 1914–1918), Rwanda was a Kingdom.

The Tutsi were the minority, making up 15% of the population. However, they had a privileged status. Tutsi kings ruled the Kingdom of Rwanda since the 15th century and held military power. While Hutus were the majority at 85% of the population, they were mostly poor peasants.

Even when Belgium colonized Rwanda after World War I, the Tutsi continued to rule the country through their Tutsi king. Later, when the king became uncooperative, the Belgians deposed him and started ruling Rwanda themselves.

In 1961, the Belgians, after their colonial rule was over, and before leaving Rwanda, put the majority Hutu in power. There were a number of marked physical differences distinguishing Tutsis from Hutus. Physically, Tutsis are slim and very tall people, usually 6 feet and taller, whereas the Hutus are typically short and stocky. Tutsis are also sophisticated, educated, and had ruled Rwanda as a kingdom for centuries.

Later, the French newspaper *Le Monde*, during the Tutsi genocide by the Hutu in 1994, wrote: "The most beautiful people in Africa, the Tutsi, are suffering."

That was why the Hutu did not give Chrys a job for many weeks, despite the fact that many hospitals in Rwanda at that time had no physicians. Even worse, Chrys was educated in the Soviet Union and had a Russian wife. The Hutu were also scared of the USSR, who were supporting military opposition forces in neighboring Congo to overthrow President Mobutu.

During its colonial rule, Belgium colonized Rwanda, Burundi, and Congo. Congo was the largest and mineral-rich country, with many metals like gold.

When Congo, after its independence, had a new nationalistic leader, Patrice Lumumba (1925–1961), President Eisenhower directly ordered the CIA to assassinate him. They did, together with Belgium and the UK.

Then, they installed their corrupt puppet Mobutu, and kept him there for 32 years while he looted Congo and became the richest man in Africa. During his reign, Mobutu stopped all of Congo's development. The towns, roads, railroads, bridges, and power lines that Belgium built during their colonialism decayed and disintegrated; jungles took over and grew over the areas. This devastation wrought in Congo by the Mobutu regime can even be seen today.

WHAT IS LIFE? WHAT IS HAPPINESS?

The USSR, or the Soviet Union, did not accept such an arrangement and opposed the Mobutu regime. That was why the Hutu also feared the USSR and considered me, a Russian, a dangerous entity.

All this I learned and comprehended much later. At that time, I was uninformed about the political situation, had no life experience, and was surprised to learn I represented any kind of threat to anyone, especially the Hutu.

NYANZA

One day, we received an order signed by 3 Ministers of Labor, Health, and Foreign Affairs ordering me to quit my job in Kigali immediately and follow Chrys to his place of employment. "You are a wife of a physician. Here wives of physicians do not work," the order cited.

The next morning, a pickup truck appeared at our new home with a driver and 2 other men inside. We put 2 items (a baby crib and a gas cooker) into the pickup truck, climbed onto the top of the truck with our infant child, and headed to the small village, Nyanza, located 90 kilometers from Kigali. Nyanza had a hospital that served many small villages in a 5–15 kilometers radius. Chrys was the only physician there.

Near Nyanza was a Catholic college run by Catholic priests from Belgium. I asked the college administration if I could teach math and physics there, but they turned me down, as they knew our story.

ESCAPE FROM RWANDA TO KENYA

Then 3 months after we had arrived, an important dignitary arrived in Nyanza. He was the United Nations' Medical Director for all of East Africa.

He was also a Russian physician and brought a secret communiqué to us, a warning message from underground organizations responsible for saving people from political prosecutions.

The message conveyed that their trusted spy, who worked for the Hutu government, reported that our names, mine and Chrys', were on a blacklist of people who were deemed to be a threat to the Hutu government and were destined to be killed any day now. The Tutsi genocide was brewing.

In order not to alarm our housemaid, who we knew was a Hutu spy, we fled to Kenya during the lunch hour with only the clothes on our backs and our child in our arms.

Later, we learned that after we escaped, Hutu men tortured our housemaid, trying to extract information about where we were supposedly hiding. They did not believe that he had no knowledge about our escape. He died 4 days later.

The following Sunday, Chrys' family and some of our friends and supporters performed memorial services in church in our memory. They were sure that the Hutu had killed us. That was typical. Thousands of Tutsis and some progressive Hutus were disappearing regularly, never to be seen again, and the Western press kept silent.

WHAT IS LIFE? WHAT IS HAPPINESS?

The 1st genocide of the Tutsi people took place in Rwanda in 1959. The Hutu government attempted to wipe out the Tutsi minority. After that, throughout the 1960s, the Hutu government launched murderous attacks against the Tutsi, to stomp out any opposition. It resulted in a mass exodus of 400,000 Tutsis into neighboring countries, such as Burundi, Congo, Uganda, Tanzania, and Kenya.

Then in 1994, the Hutu launched another Tutsi genocide, killing close to 1 million Tutsi. The Western world did not interfere; it just idly watched everything from the sidelines.

As for Chrys, why in the world, after graduating from the USSR and being a Tutsi, did he decide to go back to Rwanda, when none of his high school classmates did?

After his classmates finished their education in the USSR or in any of the other European countries, they all went to Burundi, Congo, Uganda, or Tanzania. No one went back to Rwanda to face certain death at the hands of Hutus.

Chrys' return could only be attributed to his naïveté, youth, and indeed ignorance. He did not think that he in any way represented a threat to the Hutu. He left Rwanda at a young age. He had not lived there for the last 12 years from the time he returned. He had attended a boarding school in Burundi, and then was a student at Brussels' Medical University in Belgium. From Brussels, he went to the USSR, learned Russian, and finished a medical university in Odessa.

He probably got advice from his father that Rwanda was safe. His father was a businessman and had prosperous businesses in different parts of Rwanda, and had learned to live with the Hutu. His adopted son was a Hutu and occupied a very important post, he was a Supreme Court Judge.

But Chrys was wrong, and he put our lives at risk. We survived by a stroke of luck that came from several international underground, and Red Cross organizations. They knew more about our danger than we did.

They saved our lives by sending us a messenger that did not arouse the Hutu's suspicions, a dignitary—the United Nations Medical Director for all East Africa, a Russian physician. During his visit to Nyanza and his secret warning message to us, we became informed and these organizations initiated and arranged our secret escape from Rwanda.

IN KENYA

We escaped to Nairobi, the capital city of Kenya, without a visa. The French Consulate met us at the Nairobi airport and took us under his diplomatic protection. However, 3 weeks later, when we went and asked the Immigration Department for a visa to stay in Kenya, we were denied. A red-haired British was angrily jumping up and down, giving us some sort of lecture.

I did not know one word of English and had no idea what he was talking about but recognized one word—"communists." That is what he called us and refused our visas.

After Kenya became independent from British colonial rule in 1964, Jomo Kenyatta became President and ruled Kenya for the next 20 years. Even though Kenya became independent, in reality, the British continued ruling Kenya as it was still a colony.

There were many instances when Kenya's young specialists, who graduated from the USSR and the Eastern European universities, were not allowed to enter Kenya upon their arrival back home.

At Nairobi airport, they were put on the next airplanes available and deported to any other country across the globe. Some spent days travelling in the air.

LIVING IN TANZANIA

Tanzania ended up giving us visas, and we arrived in Dar es Salaam ("Safe Port" in Arabic), a capital city. Tanzania was different. It had a progressive leader, President Julius Nyerere, known as Mwalimu or teacher in Kiswahili, who had an aspiration to build an African socialist society based on the Swahili concept of "Ujamaa" (village).

Chrys was immediately accepted into an internship program for medical doctors. He knew English very well. He received a small room in the intern's residence, free food and uniform, and a small stipend of $100 per month. He was on hospital duty 24/7 and came to see our toddler son and me on Sundays for 3–4 hours.

As for me, I faced many monumental problems and challenges. One was a new language. Rwanda was a Belgian colony, and French was their official language that I knew well. Tanzania was a former British colony, and its official language was English, a language I did not know. Another problem was finding a place to live, when we had no money. Luckily, Mr. John Bosco, a member of a refugee organization, came to see us in the motel. Out of the goodness of his heart, he took me and our son to live with him. He had a small 2 bedroom house in Kinondoni.

MY LIFE IN KINONDONI

Kinondoni was a huge suburb, the most populated district of Dar es Salaam. Tens of thousands of small, look-alike 2-bedroom houses for the Tanzanian middle class were built by Germany as economic aid to Tanzania. Each house, besides a living room and 2 bedroom, had a small yard with a water basin in the middle. At the end of the yard was another small structure consisting of a shower room, toilet, room for a kitchen, and a small room for a housemaid. In Muslim tradition, a concrete fence, 5 feet in height, was wrapped around the yard.

The bedroom Mr. John gave me was small, with only 2 pieces of furniture in it. One was an old single bed that had broken metal springs supporting a mattress; the other was a child's crib with a mosquito net. That was it. Not even a chair. I had no air conditioner, no fan, TV, radio, or telephone. The weather was always hot and humid with temperatures hovering around 100° Fahrenheit, and humidity was 100%.

My child and I were living off the small $100 stipend that Chrys received each month. Monthly rent for a 1-bedroom apartment in Dar es Salaam at that time was $300 or more.

I was cut off from the world and wrote letters to my relatives and friends in Odessa, asking them to send me Russian-English books so I could start learning English as soon as possible. They arrived 2 months later. With gusto I descended on these books to learn English so I could get back to work and life.

LESSONS IN ENGLISH
Irish Matron Cara, a director of a nursing school, asked her assistant, Miss Frica, a British lady who knew some French, to give me some lessons in English. According to her status, she lived in a big mansion alone on Ocean Drive alongside the Indian Ocean and had an old Volkswagen Beetle. Miss Frica was a spinster who had never been married.

After a few lessons, she became very curious to see how I really lived. She knew that I was living in Kinondoni, the only white woman among many Africans, so she offered me a lift to my home. There she saw for herself my meager living situation.

Amazed at how I lived, the next time she saw me she asked, "How do you feel about living in Kinondoni? You are the only white woman in an all African neighborhood, when in Odessa you lived a privileged life. You had a prestigious engineering job, a new condo, all in the beautiful city of Odessa that some tourists compare to Paris?"

I was surprised by her question. I did not even notice my meager living conditions. I was focused on my one and only objective, to learn English. Learn English as quickly as possible and go back to work and into an exciting life that was passing me by.

I answered her question, "Our situation is just a temporary one. We had the best education in the world. We are young, and our lives are all ahead of us."

The following week, I went to Miss Frica to continue my English lessons. She did not open the door. I knew she was at home; her Volkswagen was parked in her driveway. I understood that after seeing how I lived, Miss Frica's British status dictated that it was beyond her British standard to associate with me, a person with a very poor living status.

PROGRESS: A JOB IN DAR ES SALAAM
I continued to teach myself English from 6 a.m. in the morning to midnight, using a crude method that I designed myself. And 4 months later, I had learned English and got my 1st job. Before that though, I went to the Tanzanian Ministry of Education to have them evaluate and approve

my BSCE diploma, or Bachelor of Science in Civil Engineering from the USSR. That was: to certify its equivalence to an English diploma.

At the Ministry, a board made up of British men looked and examined my diploma (it was translated to English by the USSR Embassy). One of them made his own rules and regulations and announced their verdict: "You are probably an economist, not an engineer." With those words, he rejected my diploma and handed it back to me.

By this time, I was a veteran in how to handle perilous events and situations and did not panic after my diploma was rejected. No I wasted any time thinking about it. After walking a few blocks, I saw a construction site and started reading a big billboard next to it.

It was an advertisement about who designed the building and who was building it. I asked a constructions manager for help, to give me some names of the best and the largest engineering design companies in Dar es Salaam. One of the names he gave me was "Sarda Engineering Company." It was an Indian company, and I went directly to it.

I asked to see the owner, Mr. Sarda, and asked him for a job. His 1st question was: "Was your diploma approved by the Ministry of Education?" "No," I replied. "Then, I can do nothing for you," he stated. Things were beyond his control, he emphasized it by wildly opening his arms. "What about a draftsman job?" I pressed him. "A draftsman is all right," he said. "When do you want to start?" "Tomorrow," I responded. I was happy and exited.

AT LAST: LIFE GAVE ME A BREAK
So, I started work as a draftsman and poured my heart and mind into my new job. Seeing my progress and enthusiasm, a chief engineer started giving me engineering and architectural jobs as he did to all the male engineers in the company. I did them all and even better than some of the males.

Then, approximately 3 months later, I got a break. A famous local man came to our bureau to design his private villa. He was Mr. Songambili, a famous local boy, who did very well for himself. He was educated in the UK and became the Minister of Railways and Transportation.

He was a charismatic man and a newly minted millionaire. Tanzanians were proud of him. Also, he was a Muslim and had 4 wives. Mr. Sarda, without thinking, blundered. He assigned the design of his villa to me. When Mr. Songambili found that I was a woman, he was offended and humiliated.

But Mr. Sarda was an expert in public relations and manipulations. He knew how to get out of any difficult situation, and this one was no exception. Ashamed at the thought of losing such a famous client, in a few seconds he found a solution.

He told Mr. Songambili, "All right. I am sorry. My sincere apologies to you. It was my mistake. You can choose any male engineer you'd like to design your villa. Furthermore, I will not charge you for the design.

"But, before that, please do me a personal favor. Talk to Alla and find out her capabilities." Puzzled, Mr. Songambili curiously agreed. In a hurry, I was ushered into a meeting room with him.

We talked for about 40–50 minutes about his estate and what he wanted in his villa. I gave him several suggestions on how his contemporary villa design would look and at the same time meet his large family needs. The result was great. Now he wanted only me to design his villa. I did.

Then, I made copies of these drawings and calculations, attached my BSCE diploma and headed back to the Ministry of Education asking them again to approve my diploma. As soon as the same board made up of British men saw the name Songambili on my drawings, they approved my diploma without any questions.

WORKING FOR THE MINISTRY OF "COMWORKS," AN INTERNATIONAL ENGINEERING COMPANY

Now I did not want to go back to work for Mr. Sarda at the Sarda Engineering Company. He exploited me and took advantage of my situation. Even though I was doing the same job as all the other male engineers, he continued paying me the same small starting salary as if I was still a draftsman.

My dream was to work for the Ministry of Communications, Transport, Labor and Work (or "Comworks" for short), an International Engineering Company where hundreds of engineers, architects, and technicians from all over the world were designing all kinds of superstructures for Tanzania.

I was hired, but, not as an equal to the male engineers. I received no 2-year contract, no United Nations salary, no 30-days of vacation each year, and no free furnished housing. Furthermore, I had to prove myself and demonstrate that I could do the same job as all the other male engineers.

For that, I was given an exam: to design a 4-story reinforced concrete administrative building. As usual, I focused on it and poured my mind and heart into it.

Then, 4–5 weeks later, a chief engineer came to inspect what I had done. He was so impressed and excited when he saw my drawings that he grabbed my drawings from the boards and ran with them to the Director of Comworks, a British. Immediately, I was given a United Nations contract for 2-year, the same salary as my male counterparts, 30-days paid vacation, and later we received a 2-story furnished and free of charge new townhouse.

Soon, I was also promoted. A chief engineer took me into his office to design his pet projects with him; he was Ozren Seculic, a famous engineer from Zagreb, the former Yugoslavia.

We bought a bright new car, a Ford Escort. Then 1 month later, Chrys finished his internship at Muhimbili Hospital and was given a position in a small hospital located in one of the small villages in the Arusha region, about 500 kilometers from Dar es Salaam.

That was an astonishment to both of us. That meant I had to quit my dream job in Dar es Salaam and follow him, as if it was in Rwanda. Our ignorance was not a blessing; we were so naive and inexperienced at life that we never saw this coming.

However, my Ministry of Comworks learned about Chrys' assignment and asked the Ministry of Health to give Chrys a position here, in Dar es Salaam, so I could continue working for Comworks. Plus, they could not terminate my 2-year binding contract that I had signed with them. The Ministry of Health agreed.

They gave Chrys a position in Muhimbili Hospital by transferring an Indian physician from Muhimbili Hospital to Chrys' place in the Arusha region. Tanzania, like the rest of the world, had a socialized medical system and free medical care. Physicians were usually assigned to work where there was a need for them, not where they wanted to work.

OUR LIFE IN DAR ES SALAAM

At last all our problems were behind us and life was great. Dar es Salaam was blooming and booming. President Nyerere's leadership attracted foreign aid and foreign specialists from all over the world. Nationalist and socialist, he welcomed help from all countries, regardless of their system or affiliation.

Dar es Salaam had over 100 foreign embassies and different missions. Embassy parties and foreign concerts were now common in the city. There was an International Film Festival for several weeks, where I saw the movie *Doctor Zhivago* for the first time.

Some embassies also had cultural centers. In the American cultural center, I saw the film *Psycho* by Alfred Hitchcock for the 1st time.

Many countries were competing with each other to show their status, culture, and economic strength in the form of economic aid to Tanzania. For example, Germany built "Kinondoni," a suburb in Dar es Salaam built of hundreds of thousands of houses for the growing Tanzanian middle class.

The Chinese were building a railway between the Dar es Salaam port and Zambia, to bring copper from Zambia to

WHAT IS LIFE? WHAT IS HAPPINESS?

Dar es Salaam's port on the Indian Ocean, for export to Europe. Kenya's *Weekly News* newspaper called this Chinese railway "Communist Aid."

The USA did not want China to outperform them in regards to economic aid, so they started building a highway right next to the railway the Chinese were building. It seemed that Americans thought that copper needed alternative transportation, such as a highway, and could not solely rely on the Chinese railway.

What if something happened to the railway? It could breakdown, derail, be sabotaged—then the export of copper would stop. So they decided the export of copper needed alternative transportation, such as a highway, where it could easily be moved by trucks.

In full view and for all to see, the competition between the Americans and Chinese started. Who would finish first? Which system was better, capitalism or socialism? Who was going to triumph? The international media had a blast and field day reporting on the situation. Almost every day, at least 1 major Dar es Salaam newspaper reported the progress of the competition in pictures. Chinese workers, who were building the railway, lived simple lives below their means. Workers lived in railroad wagons with 30–40 people in each one. As soon as they laid down 1–2 km of rail, they moved their wagons ahead of the newly built tracks and at that point put their red colored Chinese flag with 5 stars on it—1 large star and 4 smaller ones—in the ground.

Americans were on Chinese hills, building right near their highway, also staking their stars and stripes (i.e. their flag) in the ground to indicate their progress. They had a hard time keeping up thought.

During that time, between 1968–1970, the 1st Tanzanian woman was running for vice president position. Muslims comprised 25% of Tanzanians. Muslim women started demonstrating seeking equal opportunity with Muslim men.

One Sunday, the city of Dar es Salaam and its surrounding suburbs of 1 million were paralyzed. Tens of thousands of Muslim women holding palm fronds had marched through the streets of Dar es Salaam singing and carrying placards.

They were asking for equality, the ability to have 4 husbands as Muslim men could have 4 wives.

NOTHING LASTS FOREVER

Nothing lasts forever or is taken for granted and neither was our good life. Soon our lives were threatened again. Rwanda's Hutu government discovered that not only were we alive, but we were living and doing well in Tanzania. Rwanda's Hutu President Gregoire Kayibanda (1961–1973) asked the Tanzanian President Julius Nyerere directly to extradite us "criminals" back to Rwanda for prosecution for our "2 crimes."

Our 1st "crime" was that "6 patients died" after Chrys "abandoned them after operations" and escaped from Rwanda. Our 2nd crime was that we "stole" $40,000 from the Rwandan government. These accusations were false and we had planned our escape around these possible accusations. Chrys stopped operating on patients 2–3 weeks before our escape. All his patients recovered and were discharged from the hospital.

As for the $40,000 that we "stole," no one believed it, and at that time that was a huge sum of money in Rwanda. We did not work for the Rwandan government. Rwanda's currency was Rwandese franks and not the dollar. Only some international banks in Kigali carried dollars for tourists to exchange.

Chrys worked in a government hospital, but there was a director in charge of money and operations. Health care was free and the hospital's budget was meager, just enough to pay the salaries of its employees, and all in Rwandese franks.

The Red Cross intervened and gave $40,000 to the Rwanda government. To hide us from extradition, the Red Cross transported me and my son in a jeep to a monastery located 80–90 kilometers from Dar es Salaam during the night.

They did not take Chrys; he was too toxic to be together with us, and the Red Cross feared they could not save him.

He was a Tutsi, and the Hutu wanted to prosecute him for "the death of 6 patients."

When on the other hand, I was a woman, a Russian, with 1 child and was pregnant with a 2nd. There was some mercy for me in such a situation. The Red Cross was sure that they could save me and my children, but they were doubtful they could save Chrys.

Our case was given to the Office of the Vice President of Tanzania to handle. They interviewed Chrys several times and some other people who knew us. After 1 week, they concluded that we were innocent and refused to extradite us back to Rwanda for prosecution.

ON THE RUN AGAIN—FROM TANZANIA

It was clear to us that Rwanda's Hutu government's lust for our blood did not stop there. Now they knew where we lived and would definitely try again to get rid of us using different methods. Furthermore, what was going to happen to us if the Tanzanian government changed overnight in a coup d'état, as was often an occurrence throughout the African continent?

We had to leave Tanzania as soon as possible. Where would we run? What country would take us and protect us?

The Soviet Union government policy, we learned, always took the side of other governments, not individuals. They wanted to keep good relationships with foreign governments. So we chose the USA. There, we learned, laws were designed to protect individuals.

OUR USA VISAS

During my lunch hour, I stopped at the USA Consulate to get preliminary information on how to get a visa and what was involved. To my surprise, without asking me any questions or identification, they handed me a small form to fill out. That was a visa. Later, I learned that we had come to the USA on a "brain drain" visa that the USA was giving to talented foreign engineers, scientists, and physicians.

I worked with one American engineer; he knew me very well. And, I assumed, he gave very favorable recommendation about me, as a woman Russian engineer, to his embassy. During the Cold War, both countries were spying on each other heavily. That was why the USA Consulate did not ask me any questions or for identification. I suspect that they knew more about me than I knew about myself.

I was lucky with the USA visa. But the American Consulate reminded me that I was a Soviet Union citizen and must ask the USSR Embassy to give me permission to go to the USA.

There were also other barriers to our departure, and we still could not leave Tanzania on short notice. I had signed a 2-year binding contract with the Ministry of Comworks which was going to expire at the end of the year. If I terminated my contract, I would have to pay the penalty of 8 months of my salary, plus other termination penalty fees.

We did not have that amount of money—we had spent all our money buying an expensive new car, Ford Escort, and I had helped my grandma Anna in Odessa.

Just a few months before, there was a USSR trade ship from Odessa anchored in Dar es Salaam seaport. One of the crew members was my grandma's neighbor. I took this opportunity to help my grandma, and sent all our savings to my grandma through this neighbor.

As for Chrys, to be able to practice medicine in the USA, he had to pass a 3-day ECFMG final exam (Educational Commission for Foreign Medical Graduates) in the American Embassy in Dar es Salaam. The ECFMG exam was a requirement for all physicians who graduated from medical schools outside the USA and Canada. Chrys was brilliant; he studied evenings and nights for the exam and passed it.

Soon, he received several invitations from hospitals in the USA and in Canada to complete his internship there. We chose Baltimore, Maryland. It was a seaport and reminded me of my native town, a seaport Odessa on the Black Sea.

Chrys' internship in the USA was starting soon, in June. But my contract with the Ministry of Comworks expired at the end of December.

WHAT IS LIFE? WHAT IS HAPPINESS?

I made a decision, telling Chrys, "Go, go, do not wait for me and the children. At least you will be safe." Then, I borrowed money from my friend Maria to buy him a suit, travel bag, and plane ticket to Baltimore, Maryland. Chrys also owed taxes to the Tanzanian government. For that, I asked my Ministry to transfer his taxes to me and every month to deduct it from my salary.

He had no contract with the hospital, and having a tax-free paper, he left Tanzania in May. And I was left alone in a foreign country with 2 small children—the youngest was 6 months old—and with a huge work responsibility.

THE SOVIET UNION REFUSES PERMISSION TO GO TO THE USA

With Chrys gone, I turned my attention to myself and my problematic situation. I went to the Soviet Union Embassy and spoke directly to the Ambassador, asking him to grant me permission to go to the USA. He thought that I was joking.

He was not going to risk his job for one Soviet citizen—me—and flatly refused. There was a Cold War between the 2 countries. Both countries forbade their citizens to even travel to the other country, let alone go and live there. The USSR was branded by the West as an "Iron Curtain."

The Soviet Union did not allow its citizens to travel to other foreign countries even as tourists on vacation. All of that was forbidden, especially to enemy #1, the USA. To go to another foreign country, one had to defect, which was an international scandal, propaganda event, and news extravaganza.

For example, in 1934, a black American singer, Paul Robinson, defected to the USSR. For many years the USSR used his defection as propaganda against the West.

Then, in 1961, Rudolf Nureyev was the 1st Soviet ballet defector; he defected in Paris. In 1970, ballerina Natalia Makarova, when on a foreign tour, defected to London; and in 1974, Mikhail Baryshnikov defected to Canada.

In my case, the year was 1970 when I asked the USSR for permission to go to the USA, during a time when travel was forbidden and the environment between the 2 countries was hostile and suspicious. At the same time, it was the last thing I wanted to ask some international organizations to help me with—to go to the USA, and in doing so, embarrass the USSR.

Then Chrys, who was already in the USA, wrote a letter directly to the Foreign Ministry in Moscow giving them an inventory of our life-threatening events in Africa.

He also emphasized my difficulties living in a foreign country, Tanzania, alone with 2 small children. At the end of his letter, he asked Moscow's Foreign Ministry a question: would they want their wives to be in my position?

I assumed that Moscow, in my case, was afraid of bad international publicity and ordered the Soviet Ambassador in Tanzania to grant me permission go to the USA.

MEETING MISS FRICA AGAIN

I met Miss Frica again during an International Film Festival in Dar es Salaam. Happy to see her, I ran up to her with my open arms, greeting her, "Hi, Miss Frica, I am so glad to see you again." Coldly she looked past me and ignored me completely.

Embarrassed, I looked for support from my friend Maria, who was with me and witnessed this incident. Maria reassured me: "Miss Frica is very jealous of you. You know why? Because you achieved in just 1 year more that she did in all her lifetime."

Indeed, this time my living status had changed 180 degrees since the last time I had seen Miss Frica. I had gone from my poor, meager life in Kinondoni, which Miss Frica saw that had made her feel ashamed to even associate with me.

Today I was an accomplish engineer. I had learned English and was back to my engineering profession working with hundreds of male engineers, architects, and technicians from all over the world. I was the only woman engineer there.

Everyone was impressed with my work. When the presidential lodge at Lake Duluti came to our company to design the lodge, I was chosen to design it.

We had received a new, furnished, and free 2-story townhouse. I drove a new car, Ford Escort—while Miss Frica still was driving her old Volkswagen, and I had my 2nd child. Chrys already was in the USA completing his internship.

Soon, after I finished my contract here, I was going to join him with the children in Baltimore, Maryland. That is why Miss Frica became jealous of my quick change in status, from poor to prosperous, and ignored me and my greeting.

BALTIMORE, MARYLAND, 1971: DÉJÀ VU AGAIN

I arrived in Baltimore at the beginning of 1971 with 2 small children. Chrys had rented a 2-bedroom apartment for us, but for the majority of the time he lived in the hospital, continuing his internship.

Soon, I learned the reality of life in the USA. In the USA at that time, there were not many women engineers. And those who did hold engineering degrees were lucky to get a job as secretaries in engineering companies.

I faced even more challenges: a new country, I knew only the European design (which used the metric system), and my specialty was reinforced concrete buildings. Here there were roads, bridges, and subways. Chrys was working long hours, so I was a single mom again.

MATERIALISM OR AN AMERICAN DREAM?
In the USA, I had to start all over again to prove to my male peers that I was also an engineer, equal to them. I was given challenges to design bridges, subways and a graving dock. Furthermore, I was given the most difficult and challenging projects to design. In short, what men could not design, or did not want to risk their career trying to design, they assigned to me. I had no alternative but to accept the challenges, take risks, and produce miracles, or I would lose my profession for good.

That is how and why, during my career in the USA, I designed—alone—a reinforced concrete 10-span bridge with 4 ramps over the Patapsco River, I-95, in downtown Baltimore. I found the solution how to design a spiral, and then designed this spiral for 3.5 miles of the Baltimore subway aerial structure, a design that the company considered to be the most challenging engineering design. I then received my master's degree from the Johns Hopkins University, and a doctoral degree from the George Washington University.

My skills were transferrable and I started working for health care where I created several significant innovations that brought hundreds of millions of dollars of profits per month (still continuing to this day) to HMOs and other health organizations, and hundreds of new jobs.

At the same time, Chrys finished his internship and residency, and took a 2-year fellowship in cardiology. He opened his own cardiology practice in Baltimore, Maryland.

To sum it all up, in the beginning I quickly overcame numerous challenges and difficulties and shortly thereafter, we were living the American dream. We had a modern house in upscale suburbia, our children went to the best schools including an Ivy League university.

That was how our eldest son saw our material living conditions in the USA in contrast with Africa (Rwanda and Tanzania). To him, we were prosperous and happy in the USA, while we were poor and unhappy when in Africa.

But here my personal life was empty and dull. No dreams, no excitement. Especially on the weekend. What was there to do? How should I occupy myself?

On weekends, there was only one type of pastime—malls and shopping. Feeling intellectually frustrated, I went on shopping sprees. I kept buying and buying stuff that was too expensive, that I did not need or like. I was just accumulating "stuff," filling up the house.

Many years later, I concluded that accumulated material possessions did not bring any happiness to my life. It does not make people happy. Material stuff belongs to the "quality of life" department, not to the "happiness of life" department. Money and material stuff can only improve people's quality of life, but cannot make them happy.

There are plenty of examples to reinforce my stated conclusions. The majority, if not all, rich and famous people (millionaires, movie stars, athletes, children who live on trust funds) have plenty of material things that other people do not have. They have no challenges, they do not need to struggle every day and work for a living.

The result is that they become bored and isolated. They do not know how to occupy themselves and turn to drugs, drinking, criminal mischief, divorces, and plastic surgery. All because they are unhappy. Money came easy to them. They did not work and sweat for it 24/7. They have no appreciation for money.

Wealth liberated them from physical and mental hard work. They have plenty of free time and energy. But how do you fill that and with what? They fill their boredom gap by engaging in destructive lifestyles and pursuits.

SUMMARY:
Question: What is happiness? What were the happiest years in my life? Answer: Money and material possessions can improve the quality of people's lives but will not make people happy.

Happiness is the purpose and meaning of life. To contribute to society, the world, and civilization. So later, before you die, you can look back on your life and be proud that you did not live a meaningless life. Instead, you help other people, made contributions to the society and left monuments after yourself. Do not equate material possessions, or stuff, with the meaning of life.

To reinforce the above conclusion, consider some examples (below), of the purpose and meaning of life.

EXAMPLE #1

AMERICAN MEN VOLUNTEERED TO FIGHT IN EUROPE DURING WOLD WAR II

When World War II, WWII, 1941–1945 started, the USA government asked men to volunteer in the war effort. And who were the first volunteers? Ivy League university students. Even though they came from rich or well-to-do families and lived privileged lives, these young and idealistic men volunteered for the war with dignity and honor to be the first in line to fight.

Among them were 2 future presidents of the USA: John F. Kennedy and George H. W. Bush. They knew very well that many of them would not come back home alive. And the majority of those who did return, would end up being wounded. Kennedy's brothers volunteered; the eldest brother Joseph Jr. was killed, and John F. Kennedy was wounded. George H. W. Bush was a pilot. His airplane was gunned down and burned; he survived but was wounded, yet his 2 crewmen did not survive.

Many Hollywood stars put their careers on hold to fight in the war—Clark Gable, Jimmy Stuart, Henry Fonda, Paul Newman, and Kirk Douglas, to name just a few. They were wealthy and famous. Hollywood stars earned over 300 medals and awards for their heroic actions. There were also a number of professional athletes who answered the call to serve their country.

Why did those courageous idealists leave their privileged lives behind, join the war effort, and choose to sacrifice their young or famous lives? For these war veterans, the purpose of life was to volunteer to fight Fascism and save civilization. That was a much greater purpose and meaning of life than their individual pursuits.

EXAMPLE #2

AMERICA'S GREATEST GENERATION

In the 1930s, America's Greatest Generation (journalist Tom Brokaw gave this name to the generation that lived during the Great Depression and World War II) went through depression, poverty, unemployment, and soup lines. When World War II started they actively participated in the war effort. This became known as the G.I. Generation (born 1901–1924).

Another group of the Great Generation worked at home in factories to produce ammunitions, supplies, and uniforms.

There was a shortage of food and housing, but no one noticed. They focused their energy on one common goal: to win the war.

After the war they continued contributing to the USA, building civil industries, and cheap and affordable housing and highways on a mass scale to satisfy the needs of the civilian population. Middle-class consumers were born and changed American capitalism. America now had 3 classes: the "have-all" rich capitalists, the minority; the middle class—consumers, educated and prosperous—the majority of the population; and the "have-not," the other minority.

The Greatest Generation worked for humble wages while inflation was high, but never complained. They worked tirelessly, with passion and excitement in hopes of giving a better life to their children and grandchildren.

They gave much to their country and sought little in return. That was how their collective work, stoicism, and nationalism created national wealth: houses, railroads, autos, refineries, weaponry, space programs, highways, and bridges. They created national wealth and left it all for the next generations.

EXAMPLE #3

RUSSIAN MEN

When Hitler's army invaded the Soviet Union on June 22, 1941, young Russian men were throwing their bodies under German tanks to stop their advancement on Mother

WHAT IS LIFE? WHAT IS HAPPINESS?

Russia. During the war, 1941–1945, 26.6 million Russians were killed, almost all men between the ages of 18 and 50.

They gave their lives for their motherland and for future generations. And the lucky ones who came back from the frontline were invalids, without arms, legs, and eyes, or were severely wounded and would later die shortly thereafter from these injuries.

EXAMPLE #4
RUSSIAN WOMEN

The Soviet Union won the World War II, 1941–1945. By June 1944 the Soviet Army liberated the Soviet Union, major part of Europe, and was marching on Berlin. On May 2, 1945 it concurred Berlin, and the victory was announced on May 9, 1945. But at what cost? During the 4 years of World War II, 3 years, 1941–1944, were fought on Russian soil and 26.6 million Russians perished.

The country lay in ruins. There were no superstructures, no housing, no schools, no factories, no water systems, no sanitary systems, no electricity—all were destroyed and leveled. After the war, hunger and disease descended upon the destitute and vulnerable population. Only women, old men, and children were mostly left to rebuild the ruined country.

The war produced millions of widows with small children. Millions of mothers lost their sons. And another group of women, millions of young brides-to-be, never got married or raised families because their future would-be grooms were killed in the war.

About 15 million children were orphaned, with many living semi-wild for 4 years on the streets and in ruined buildings scavenging for food and shelter to survive.

The Soviet Union government faced challenges of epic proportions. How to stop hunger and disease? How to rebuild the country and save the Russian nation? How to do all this with mostly women, old men and children?

The Soviet government found the solution—Russian women. They called on Russian women to save the nation and rebuild the destroyed country; they asked them to make extraordinary personal sacrifices so that the country could survive and the Russian nation could live.

They asked women to work 2 shifts everyday, 16 hours a day. During the day, to work on construction sites rebuilding schools, roads, and buildings, and in factories producing goods for the population and arms for the army.

Then in the evening to enter high schools, technical schools, and universities to become engineers, teachers, physicians, economists, and technicians. Women needed to receive this education as they replaced the men who were killed.

All Russian women answered the call of duty. They sacrificed and worked 2 shifts everyday. In 15–20 years they rebuilt the country, saved the Russian nation, and millions of women graduated with bachelor's and technical degrees in engineering, science, education, medicine, economics, accounting, and many technical specialties.

Women sacrificed and succeeded beyond imagination. Less than 1 generation later, Russian women outperformed their men. Every year, 75% of Russian women were graduating from universities versus 25% of men. As for teachers and physicians, more than 90% were women.

As for Western Europe, after the war, the USA established economic aid called the "George Marshall Plan" to feed the starving population and help rebuild the West European superstructures devastated by World War II. This aid was also offered to the USSR, but the USSR refused. To repeat:

□ □ □

THE MORAL OF THE STORY

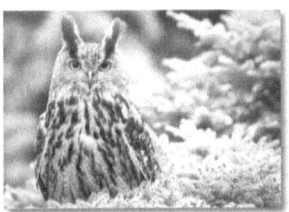

Question: What is happiness? What were the happiest years of your life? Answer: Money and material possessions can improve people's quality of life, but cannot make people happy.

Happiness is the purpose and meaning of life. To contribute to society, the world and civilization. So later, before you die, you can look back on your life and be proud that you did not live a selfish life. Instead, you made some contributions to other people and left monuments after yourself. Do not equate material possessions, or stuff, with the meaning of life.

When life has a purpose, a person elevates himself above material selfishness to a much higher level of human development, called self-actualization, as per Maslow's theory of the hierarchy of human needs.

SHORT STORY

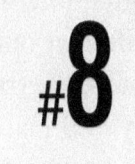

AFRICA: AN INTERRUPTED DREAM. OR, WONDERFUL LIFE DISCOVERIES IN UGANDA, RWANDA, KENYA AND TANZANIA

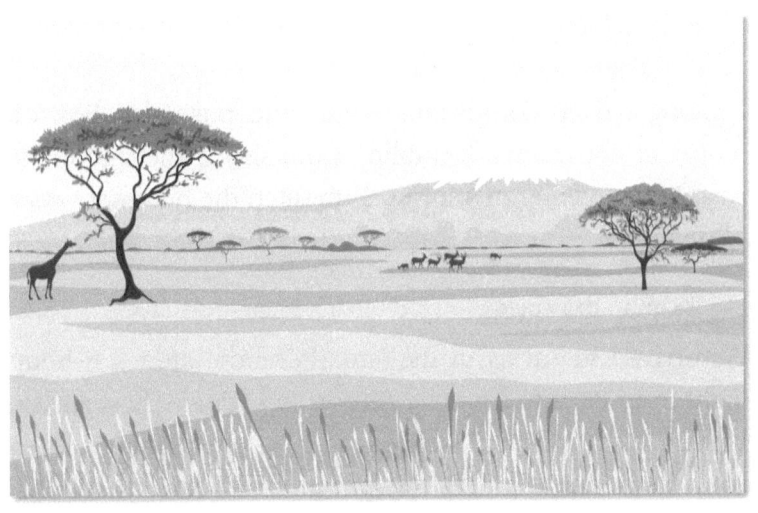

☐ ☐ ☐

Without paying much attention, I was flipping through the TV channels, and drifted at one. My heart, before my mind, had already recognized the tranquil, colorful, unique, and unforgettable scenery and reacted. Exotic acacia trees radiating clusters of white and pink spike flowers dotted a magnificent landscape. Africa! I stopped at the channel.

An avalanche of emotions, sad and warm, forced their way and flooded my body. Uncontrollable tears started running for the exit, mourning interrupted dreams, the tragic African continent, and its now crumbling civilization.

I stood up to strengthen my wobbling body. Burning in the deepest craters of my mind, now my life in Africa popped up to the surface, flooding and welcoming me, her old and trusted friend, back to Africa.

I chose a deep comfortable chair and pushed a box of tissues closer to me. Trembling from shock and fighting a rush of competing memories, I revisited the happiest years of my life in Africa.

UGANDA, ENTEBBE

We arrived in Africa in the late afternoon, after a 6-hour flight from Paris to Entebbe Airport in Uganda, East Africa. Exiting the airplane, I stepped onto a new continent. The sun was bright, the heat was pronounced, and the asphalt was soft as a thick sponge. It was my 1st rendezvous with heat and the tropical weather.

We were transferred to a nearby hotel on Lake Victoria. After the long flight, I was tired and, after dinner, immediately hit my pillow.

Sleep forgot about me and skipped my pillow but not the armies of insects outside. One army after another began tuning up their songs. At first timidly and unsure from far away, trying one tune after another.

Competing armies of new quartets appeared drumming up their songs, overpowering already singing vocalists. Soon, all the armies of singers joined together in unison and filled the night. I heard nothing but the loud and powerful singing of insects, hundreds of thousands, or millions of them, testing their vocal cords.

Unaccustomed to such nightly serenades, guarding myself from the unknown and unexpected, I tuned up my senses to full volume and the insects' songs magnified.

In the end, I had no alternative but to get used to them; they serenaded me into deep sleep. I was on the African continent, mysterious and exotic and over 5,000 kilometers away from my home.

When I awoke, the first morning sunrays were beating through the shuttered wooden windows slats, skewed at 45 degrees. I assumed it was around 6 a.m. I had read before that near the equator, the sunrise is at exactly at 6 a.m. and the sunset at 6 p.m., pronto, every day, every season, 12 months a year. Half of the sun was still buried behind the horizon.

Curious, I opened a door to the patio and stepped into a huge field of planted flowers, very familiar to me, tall zinnias, displaying rainbow cascades of different colors.

Instinctively, to make me feel comfortable in this unknown environment, my mind retrieved previous zinnias memories and brought me back to my childhood days. When I was a child, to reach an orchard full of apple, pear, peach, and cherry trees, I needed to walk a narrow path. On both sides of the path grandma planted flowers, tall zinnias.

Feeling nostalgic, I continued crossing the zinnia plantation, and feeling happy as a child. I had no fear or hesitation now. At the end of the plantation, fencing the zinnia field, was an opening among huge exotic trees.

I walked directly into another surprise—Lake Victoria. I sat on the bank and looked at the lake. I already knew that it was the largest fresh water lake in Africa and the principal source of the Nile Basin.

My introduction to Lake Victoria was like a scene in some movies, when a sudden calm was replaced by a raging hurricane and viewers' emotions were thrown from one extreme to another.

WHAT IS LIFE? WHAT IS HAPPINESS?

For many miles I was alone. Around me, as far as the horizon, there was no sight or sound of civilization. I saw no animals, heard no birds, only the silence and the calm lake's majestic, divine, and surreal surface. The lake was on this earth for thousands of years. It had witnessed the birth, rise, fall, and disappearance of many civilizations.

I did not know for how long in time I was lingering there melting into the natural world of Lake Victoria. What a natural life and discovery I walked into!

RWANDA, NYANZA

Before coming to Rwanda, I had read that it was the most beautiful country in Africa. It had been called Africa's Switzerland, or a country of a "thousand rolling hills."

We arrived in Nyanza from Kigali, where Chrys received his assignment to work in the main hospital. Nyanza was a royal capital; Rwanda's kings were living there. We got a house, the mansion, of the former Belgian governor who lived there during the colonial era.

Today, the mansion was run down. No one had lived there for some time and, upon our arrival, we spent the rest of the day busily cleaning just a few rooms from insects, dust, and spider webs for the night.

The morning came. I opened a window to get some fresh air and was frozen from all future actions. In front of me was a panoramic view of the earth's eternity in its full glory.

Rolling hills, like an uninterrupted rhapsody, majestic and untouchable, covered by dark green flora, invited me to get a glance into their ancient life.

A fog, not yet evaporated by the sun, in waves of different thickness, was nourishing the life on the hills with moisture. For millions of years, these ancient hills were living here, rolling from one elevation onto another, and gracefully projecting their undeniable eternity.

What is the length of a human life in comparison to the ancient life of the rolling hills? Shocked by the contrast between a short human life and the life of the hills, I questioned my existence as a human.

It seemed to me that a human life mimicked the life of the ancient hills. In mass, hills were enormous and if not immeasurable, where one human being's weight was just a small particle of sand grain in the universe.

The hills were millions of years old and continue living forever. The length of 1 human life was a short, 40–80 years. The hills underwent many changes together with the universe, just as a human being also goes through many physical and mental changes in the 40–80 years of his or her life.

A human life started from a seed, developed into a fetus in a mother's womb, then burst into outside life as a baby. The baby grew into a child, a teenager, and then an adult. The process also changes a human intellect. Then in the end, a human life exhausts itself and dies, is buried and dissolves to join other forms, as a contributor to the earth's eternal life, or the earth's endless cycle of life.

I extracted myself from the window only to find that a huge amount of tears, for some times, had been running down my cheeks onto my clothes. My instincts and emotions were far ahead of my thinking. They recognized the importance of my discovery of eternity and acted upon it. At once, my human death and any fears regarding it became unimportant.

For several minutes I was admitted into the eternal life of the rolling hills. I was privileged to see what few have seen before me: the unforgettable, divine, and beautiful nature that is imprinted in my mind and heart forever. From that point on, I never feared for my life, nor was I ever scared of death.

TROPICAL RAINS

Rwanda is only a few degrees south of the equator, but it has a relatively moderate climate, 75°F–55°F, thanks to the high altitudes of its hills. There are 2 rainy periods. One is in March–May and another in September–December.

Tropical rains in Rwanda are unforgettable, forceful, loud, and spectacular. When the sun is shining at its brightest level, suddenly, without any warning, the rain originates in one faraway point and, like a tornado with a crushing noise, quickly moves toward one. Closer and closer. It is here.

Like an army of vicious invaders, the rain lashes out at everything standing in its path. The sky opened and for a short while the water poured out in a tremendous display of Mother Nature's power. Then it stopped as suddenly as it started.

The sun was back, shining again as if nothing happened. Was it my imagination, or a tropical rain? Look around. Many small water ponds appeared everywhere, reminding me that indeed a rain shower had occurred here, and the ground had no time to absorb the water yet.

I could smell the fragrant oil from the soil and flora brought out by the rain. Trees, bushes, flowers, and grass came back to life, bursting into sparkling green colors, happy and grateful for the life nourishment the tropical rain had supplied. Now it was time for tourists to take some picturesque photographs.

POPULATION DENSITY

Escaping from Rwanda to Kenya on a small plane, I sat glued to a window, sadly looking down, knowing that I had probably seen Rwanda for the last time. Below, a stretch of hundreds of hills of different heights covered the landscape.

Between hills, valleys were overpopulated by small typical Rwandese round huts made from clay bricks each topped

WHAT IS LIFE? WHAT IS HAPPINESS?

by a cylindrical cone made from straws. A small piece of land, probably about 1/4, or 1/3 of an acre, was left around each hut. Everywhere cone huts, like on a chessboard, were located next to each other.

Africans had very large families, with a typical size of 6–10 children. Where did they get land to grow enough food for such big families? I wondered. Rwanda was the most densely populated country in Africa.

In 1967, it had a population of 3.4 million and a density of 335 people per square mile. Before the genocide of the Tutsi in 1994, the total population grew to 5.7 million and the density increased to 562 people per square mile. In 2012, as per Rwanda's census counts, the population increased to 11.5 million, and the density to 1,126 people per square mile.

In other words, in the last 45 years the total population and density in Rwanda exploded over 3.3 times.

Where had they gotten the land for such a population explosion? By moving into the jungle, cutting tropical trees and bushes, killing and displacing wild animals, and reclaiming jungles to plant agricultural crops. There are not enough jungles left to convert into agricultural land.

Overpopulation and a scarcity of land in Rwanda, as some West European newspapers cited later, was one major factor that contributed to Rwanda's genocide in 1994 that killed close to 1 million Tutsi, the majority of the Tutsi population.

NAIROBI, KENYA

Our escape to Nairobi from Rwanda was, at the beginning, a pleasant bonus. Nairobi was a beautiful contemporary city, a safari capital of Africa, and a Mecca for adventurers. Flamboyant flowering trees, heavy and impressive, with crimson and purple colored blossoms, were spectacular.

The city was lost among a breathtaking wealth of flowering trees, shrubs, flowers, bright sun, and tropical weather. Indigenous exotic trees and plants glowed in the riot of color, invigorating life like no other city I know.

Calling attention to them, stood out hundreds of types of different acacias, flowering a dense cluster of pink and white colors and imprinted unforgettably beautiful scenery in the minds of many visitors. After 1 month, we said good-bye to Nairobi, after the British colonial establishment, which continued to rule Kenya after independence, refused to give us a visa. We headed to Tanzania.

TANZANIA, DAR ES SALAAM

We lived in Tanzania for almost 3 years. At the beginning in Kinondoni, then in Illala. Both were huge suburbs of Dar es Salaam built by Europeans as economic aid for the Tanzanian middle class. I observed and learned from exposure to the local life around me. Some examples and episodes are below.

"A THIEF IS COMING." OR, IN SWAHILI, "MWIZI NAKWENDA."

Local people are afraid of thieves and are very protective of their meager possessions. Once they hear or see one, the whole neighborhood gets involved, running after the thief, yelling, and beating drums to alert others to join them in the chase, yelling "Mwizi nakwenda! Mwizi nakwenda!" while throwing stones at the thief and trying to capture him.

I had many personal experiences with "mwizis." They knew that I was a white woman living in an all-black neighborhood, and during the night I was alone with my small son. Mr. John Bosco (the owner of the house) was working as manager at the hotel Kilimanjaro. He was a bachelor and, after visiting some night bars, would come home to sleep early in the morning; his job started at noon.

My helper, a teenage boy named Nikko, would sleep in his small room at the end of the courtyard and never woke up from my screams. Chrys, my then husband, lived in the Muhimbili Hospital in the interns' quarter, completing his internship for physicians.

I was lucky, I always woke up from the noise, as a mwizi, to get into the house, had to climb a 5-foot fence and once inside the yard, stepped on the gravel. Usually, as soon as I heard him, I started yelling: "Mwizi nakwenda!"

That was enough to send terrifying signals to the mwizi. At once he recognized the danger that he had been discovered and should expect all consequences when the whole neighborhood started running after him to capture and punish him. The thieves always run.

"BEANS AND PANCAKES." OR, IN SWAHILI "MAHARAGE AND CHAPATI"

Maharage and Chapati are a typical breakfast of Tanzanians. In Kinondoni, every morning, our son on his tricycle would pedal directly into local African living rooms, where they were eating breakfast.

They loved him and happily made a place for him in their circle, and soon he would be eating breakfast with them like a family member. They affectionately called him "Fideli." He spoke Swahili perfectly and even knew some Swahili jokes.

When we bought a new car, a Ford Escort, our son liked to stand up, looking around from the sunroof while I was driving. When they saw him all the neighborhood children would run alongside escorting our car and yelling "Fideli nakwenda," ("Fideli is coming") for miles.

Later, when we moved into a new townhouse in Illala, early in the morning, before we parents woke up, our son would be up and on the balcony. There he stopped and questioned any adult who happened to be passing near by, yelling out to him: "Nakweda yko wapi wewe Bwana?" ("Where are you going, sir?") Sir, the Tanzanian adult, would stop and become involved in a long conversation with him. Africans love children and take them seriously.

A LITTLE MONKEY LIVING IN A MANGO TREE
At the entrance to Mr. Bosco's house was a huge mango tree with a small young monkey living in it. Every morning, she would watch me leave for work, then she would enter through an open window to our bedroom, and climb into our son's crib.

At the beginning, he was afraid of her, and kept calling Nikko for help, yelling and screaming "Keniago! Keniago!" ("A clown! A clown!")

There were many small children around in our neighborhood. Each Christian family had 4–8 children, and a Muslim family had a dozen or more from 4 wives. Out of all the children around, for some reason the little monkey had chosen our child as her favorite. She liked him and if someone approached him or picked him up, she would become agitated and threatening, running around making high-pitched noises until he was back on the ground, alone.

Eventually he got used to her and would play with her. Many times I would come home and find the little monkey sitting on a sofa in our living room, chewing gum and making and pulling strings from the gum. Later, when she grew up, she left to join her troop in the nearby jungles.

BEES AND HONEY

Mr. John Bosco's house, where he, from the goodness of his heart, gave us 1 bedroom, had a small yard with orange, papaya and banana trees, and some flowering bushes. One group of bees would take nectar from flowers, regurgitate it, and deposit it into their hives; another group took the nectar and deposited it into honeycombs that they constructed above my bedroom window.

One day, the honeycombs broke down from the weight of the honey. Honey spilled out into my bedroom, disturbing thousands of bees that were angrily flying around the honey. I closed our son inside the car since the situation was dangerous. I had no alternatives but to contact a fire station in Dar es Salaam for help. Unfortunately, they used gas and exterminated all the bees.

"KENIAGO," (A "CLOWN")

Keniago was a man who came to our Kinondoni neighborhood to sell peanuts to children. To attract attention to his business, he wore a colorful mask, and so we could hear him, he tied a ring with a dozen small bells around his knee. Stamping his foot, the bells would ring, and children would pop up to the streets to buy his treat, the small bags of peanuts. The children called him Keniago.

THE MORAL OF THE STORY

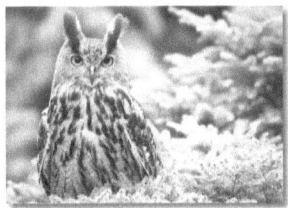

When living in Africa, I made wonderful life discoveries. They are precious gems, imprinted in my heart, nostalgically mooring memories of people and places I left far behind.

We left Africa and moved to the USA. Years later, the oil embargo of 1973–1974 devastated Africa and for a while stopped all economic development across the continent. The African dream was interrupted.

Today, my African memories keep revisiting my heart, warm and sad, reminding me about the happiest years in my life and about the crumbling now African civilization.

SHORT STORY

#9

PASSION. BELIEVE IN YOURSELF AND ACHIEVE YOUR DREAMS. AN UNEXPLAINED PHENOMENON

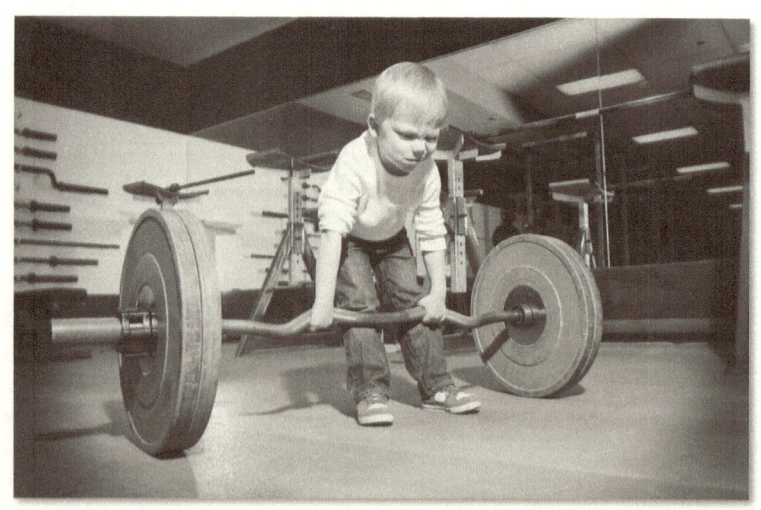

WHAT IS LIFE? WHAT IS HAPPINESS?

□ □ □

On my way to Africa, Rwanda, I was very fearful, worried, and concerned about my new life on a new continent. I prepared myself to encounter many challenging difficulties and problems associated with a new country: a foreign language, new culture, an unfamiliar environment, a different political system, new customs, laws and regulations, and even the tropical weather. When I arrived in Rwanda, none of that happened to me. Instead, a strange phenomenon[1] occurred.

From a very shy young woman with low self-esteem, who always feared speaking up to teachers, people in authority or strangers, I suddenly became as fearless as a 3-year-old child, unaware of any danger around me.

Overnight my personality was transformed and my fears disappeared. I started believing in myself to such an extent that I had no difficulties in solving all my monumental, life-threatening problems. Boldly, I was in charge of my own life and destiny.

Many rhapsodies have been written about this phenomenon by the Europeans, who arrived in Africa and experienced the same personal transformation as I did. All their fears disappeared; they became fearless and started believing in themselves.

There are many theories about this phenomenon and transformation. One theory that stood out was that all humans originated and came from Africa. Africa was the birthplace of humanity. Now we Europeans were coming back to Africa, to our roots, our origin. A powerful magnetic connection existed between the African soil and us Europeans. Africa, our ancestral birthplace, was welcoming us back home. At this home we felt secure, had no fears, and believed in ourselves.

LEARNING ENGLISH

If I am wrong, and the above theory is incorrect, then someone should explain to me how it was possible for me to learn the English language in just 4 months while in Africa. I learned English to such level that when I went to my 1st job interview, not one thought ever crossed my mind about the quality of my English.

Would an interviewer understand me, or me, him? That fear never crossed my mind. I believed that my English was very good, and that I could hold my own in any conversation. During my 1st interview, I was hired.

Never mind that before that, I had a fundamental obstacle when it came to learning foreign languages. I was an awful linguist. Learning French in school was a difficult process for me. Compared to my friends who were good linguists, I was at the bottom of the list.

Some of my friends had a gift, and quickly and easily were able to learn French. Compared to them, I had to put a lot of my energy and time into learning French. I was good in math and science, but French was an uphill battle.

WHAT IS LIFE? WHAT IS HAPPINESS?

It took me 10 years to master French. First in school, where French was a mandatory subject; then at civil engineering university where French, like any other engineering subject, was also mandatory.

MORE OBSTACLES

I had many more obstacles during the time I was learning English. We were refugees in Dar es Salaam, Tanzania. Before that, we were living in Rwanda, a French-speaking country. When the Tutsi genocide intensified, and we learned that we were on the blacklist of the Hutu government, in a hurry, we escaped from Rwanda to Tanzania, Dar es Salaam, via Kenya.

In Dar es Salaam, one member of a refugee organization gave me a small room in his 2-bedroom house to live with our infant child. The house was located in Kinondoni, a huge suburb of Dar es Salaam recently built by Germany, as foreign aid for the Tanzanian middle class.

I did not know one word of English, had no car, no telephone, no TV, no radio, no newspaper. I had no clue, no guidance, and no tips on how to self-learn English quickly. I was young, ignorant, had no wisdom, no street skills, and very little life experience. I had no one to practice my English with either. My youth and ignorance were not a blessing.

Kinondoni was located several miles from the city of Dar es Salaam. The city had a library and a university. In the university was a language course, English as a second language. I crossed out the idea to take this course. It would take a long time, 1–2 years. There was a local bus going to the city, but it was always overcrowded and unreliable. Without knowing English, I would get lost in the city, so I seldom traveled to Dar es Salaam until my 1st job interview.

I did not even notice my sub-standard life in Kinondoni; I just dwelled on the other impossible obstacles I was facing. I knew all those other difficulties were temporary.

My life was ahead of me. My passion and focus at that time was on one thing only, to learn English as soon as possible then get a job and rejoin the world. Working with other people, learning from them, and interacting with them were my goals.

My work was my life. And my life was learning, dreaming, growing, getting excited, and traveling to see the world.

I wrote a letter to my relatives and friends in Odessa in the Soviet Union, asking them to send me some Russian-English books so I could start learning English. I improvised and designed a crude learning method. Based on that method, with passion I was learning English all day and evening from 6 a.m. to midnight for 4 months.

After 4 months, a phenomenon happened: I learned English. I was so confident in my English abilities that it never even crossed my mind that my English might be an obstacle to getting a job. The only obstacle that crossed my mind was that I was a young woman engineer. Could I overcome the ignorance and prejudice in the male engineering industry to become a woman structural engineer?

The year was 1968, and there were not only no women engineers in Tanzania, but there were no women engineers in England or the USA.

The fact was, when I went to the Ministry of Education in Tanzania asking them to approve my diploma (to make it equivalent to the English Bachelor of Science in Civil Engineering, or BSCE), the Board of British men told me: "You must be an economist, not an engineer" and did not approve my BSCE diploma.

I made a discovery that learning a foreign language—in my case, English—was the most difficult subject in the world, especially compared to other subjects, for example, math, physics, or chemistry. Why? To pass an exam in hard sciences can happen due to luck, or getting easy questions that you know, or having a teacher who is easy on all the students that cannot solve all the hard science problems.

Not when learning a foreign language. With language there was only one result—you know how to compose a sentence and conduct a conversation or you do not. No one can help you and "luck" does not come into play.

Once you start speaking, your knowledge of the language is immediately exposed. An analogy could be a structural engineer who has designed a bridge in the air. All his work is exposed for all to see. If he makes even one mistake in that design, the bridge would start to crumble and collapse.

In Africa, my personality was transformed overnight from a fearful young woman with low self-esteem and who was unsure of herself, to a fearless one. I started believing in myself. Once I learned English, immediately I got the job and the rest is history, and miracles followed.

THE MORAL OF THE STORY

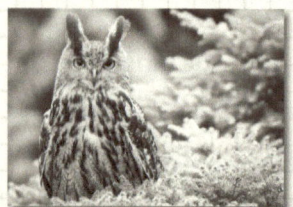

In Africa I learned to have a great passion for everything I do; without passion nothing is achievable. I always put my heart and mind into my problems. I believed in myself and miracles happened.

The same is applicable to my readers. There is nothing that you cannot do, or cannot achieve.

WHAT IS LIFE? WHAT IS HAPPINESS?

With passion[1] and enthusiasm, start believing in yourself, and the luck and miracles will follow. You will overcome all immense difficulties and achieve all your dreams.

---

[1] Phenomenon, as per Merriam-Webster's dictionary, is: an interesting fact or event that can be observed. Typically it is unusual or difficult to understand or explain in full. Passion is believing in yourself, your ideas, your cause. Passio in Latin means suffering. Emotions: there are many types that we experience in everyday life: anger, sadness surprise, happiness, fear, boredom, and frustration.

To learn about the rest of my life events in Africa, please read my other short stories in this book, "What is Happiness? What Were the Happiest Years of Your Life?" and also "Africa: an Interrupted Dream. Or, Wonderful Life Discoveries in Uganda, Rwanda, Kenya and Tanzania."

SHORT STORY #10

WHY DO AFRICANS HAVE LESS HEART DISEASE, DIABETES, AND CANCER? AND NO DEPRESSION, OSTEOPOROSIS, ARTHRITIS, OR ASTHMA?

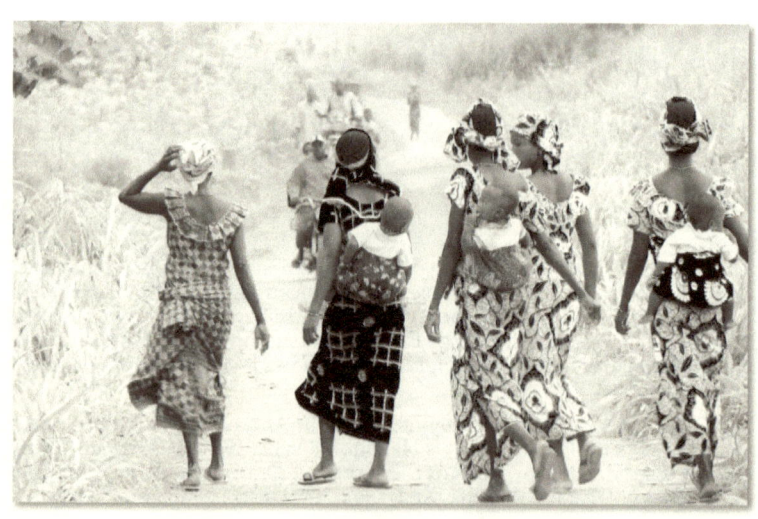

WHAT IS LIFE? WHAT IS HAPPINESS?

□ □ □

OBSERVATIONS IN RWANDA
When we arrived in post-colonial Rwanda, Central Africa, a former Belgian colony and French-speaking country, I made some observations during the 1st few weeks.

My 1st observation and question was why Africans had fewer heart disease, diabetes, cancer? And no depression, osteoporosis, arthritis, or asthma? I asked this question my then husband, Chrys, who was a physician. He did not know either.

My 2nd question was, where did African women get all their energy and strength? African women worked all day in the fields under the scorching sun, from sunrise to sunset, very often with babies on their backs, and ate only one meal in the evening.

Even then, it was just a small amount of food—no meat, no eggs, and only a cup of milk sometimes.

I could not find the answers to this riddle. With the passage of time, those questions became buried in my memories and stayed dormant for many years.

TV NEWS ABOUT "A SILENT KILLER"
In the middle of the 1990s, there was popular TV news report about a new disease, "a silent killer"—osteoporosis. At that time, I was living on the East Coast, and before

then I had never been sick, nor did I take any medication, except an occasional aspirin for a headache.

Naively I reacted to the news, thinking I probably had osteoporosis and did not know I had it. My grandmother had severe osteoporosis. Did I have her genes?

Soon I went to a newly opened Osteoporosis Institute where a university hospital in Maryland had quickly reacted to the hysteria, and in a hurry, opened the institute to the public. I found the best endocrinologist and took a bone density test. To my shock, I found I had already lost 20% of my bone density.

A physician prescribed 4 drugs: Fosamax, Provera, Premarin, and Hydrochlorothiazide. Dutifully, I took these drugs every morning believing they were reversing or stopping the rapid loss of my bones. They did, according to the test.

After 2 years, my bone loss went down to 5% from the initial 20%. Delighted and encouraged, I never missed a dose.

LIVING IN SAN FRANCISCO
I moved to San Francisco at the insistence of my eldest son to start a new life and find refuge from my divorce that had been going on for 6 years.

I was happy. For the first time in my life, I was free and did not have the 24/7 responsibilities of being a mother, housewife, employee, or, a graduate student. I sold our family home in Maryland, and the children were now adults and had graduated from college. I rented the most beautiful apartment next to the Fairmont Hotel in Nob Hill and, like a child, began discovering life around me.

Little did I know that fate had different plans in store for me. After 3 years, I started fainting, had dizziness, nausea, vertigo, a heart rate of 150–160 beats per minute, and a many more symptoms. I felt like I was dying.

To find out why, I went to numerous physicians covering my area from San Francisco all the way to San Jose. All of them gave a different diagnosis, and not one diagnosis made any sense or helped me in any way.

A BREAKTHROUGH, A CORRECT DIAGNOSIS

One day I fainted on the street and was brought to a university hospital. There, young interns felt sorry for me, but they had no clue about my illness. So they called Dr. Morley, their star professor, in the hope that he could help me. In just 5 minutes, Dr. Morley made his diagnosis: "I know why you are gravely ill. Recently there was a study published where 74 patients died with symptoms similar to yours. It is due to the side effects of the drugs you are taking. They were taking the same drugs for osteoporosis as you are. You must stop taking those drugs now." I did, and recovered.

SITE EFFECTS OF OSTEOPOROSIS DRUGS

But my immune system collapsed and opened the gate for infections that I had never heard of before. On top of that, I contracted H-pylori when I went to a dentist. I was prescribed antibiotics, but not the ordinary ones.

I took 3 sets each contained 3–4 the strongest antibiotics, but there was no progress in sight. I had no energy or strength to function. All of that time I was lying in my bed, not moving, saving energy for the next even, and the next smallest tasks.

Food gave me energy. But my stomach reacted badly to most foods, and the pain was unbearable. The main foods I ate were bananas and dry toasted bread. Exhausted and undernourished, I lost a lot of weight. I was realistic and knew that a wonder cure was remote and I, by some chance, would recover.

Soon I was going to die, I thought, and it was a matter not of if, but when. I knew the impending result once the antibiotics stopped working. The truth was that I was resigned to my fate now.

One day, I was lying in my bed feeling nostalgic. Randomly, I retrieved a section of my life from when we were living in Africa. For more than 3 years, I worked in post-colonial Africa, in Rwanda and Tanzania. There, thousands of engineers, architects, economists, teachers, physicians, technicians, and Peace Corps volunteers from all over the world had come to African countries to help them design and build new urban civilization.

WHAT WAS THE CURE TO MY ILLNESSES?
African memories, stored deep in my mind, opened the gate to a stream of information, competing for my attention. I assumed that my subconscious was on a mission, looking for only one special piece of information—a solution to how I could live and survive.

Without any effort on my part, I got a vivid answer. The sun! The sun! The solution was beaming. Now I knew why Africans had less heart disease, diabetes, cancer, and no depression, osteoporosis, arthritis, or asthma. It was because they were in the sun all day! Then I started connecting the dots between the sun and my illness.

The sun strengthen the immune system and closes the gate to all outside diseases and illnesses. African women, as I observed, worked all day, from sunrise to sunset, under the sun, plowing fields. Many of them with small children on their backs, wrapped in pieces of cloth. African women dressed in bright colored clothes to cover their bodies, except their eyes and feet.

Their heads were also covered by pieces of fabric. The sun was beaming directly into their eyes, specifically into the corners of their eyes.

REINFORCING THAT THE SUN WAS A CURE TO MY ILLNESSES

The fact was, until then, I had never been sick before even with a cold. Why? How was it possible? Had the sun been responsible for my good health? I quickly went through the inventory of my behavior and life in the USA. Before coming to the USA we choose to live in Baltimore for one reason. Baltimore was a seaport on the ocean and reminded me of my native city Odessa, a seaport and resort city on the Black Sea.

Growing up in Odessa, my best times were during the summers. Spending all day on the beach with my friends, competing to get the deepest bronzed body. The Odessa population of over 700,000 was in love with the Black Sea. There was no happier time than to spend all day lying under the sun on the beach. Going to the beach was the major activity "to do" during the summer in Odessa.

To get a place on the beach, one had to wake up early in the morning and go to the beach to claim a piece of sand. By 7:00 a.m., it would be too late. By that time the entire population of Odessa was laying on the sandy beaches, 20–30 kilometers in both directions. During the summer, the population of Odessa usually tripled in size; a lot of people from the north arrived to spend their summer on Odessa's beaches.

Old, young, locals and tourists all were there. It was a sea of bodies in swim suits, tightly packed together like sardines. To get a place between them was difficult. There were discussions, volleyball games, playing cards, as well as kiosks selling refreshments, snacks, ice cream, and cold drinks everywhere. In the evening, happy and suntanned, beachgoers returned to the city, crowding onto public transportation.

At the end of the summer, my body was dark bronze and it would take several months to fade.

When we arrived in Baltimore, I immediately checked the beach. Amazingly, it was empty. No one was walking, wandering, or sitting and dreaming, and no one was sunbathing. I missed the sun and my bronzed body.

Soon I learned that in the USA, swimming pools replaced the beach. So, I hit the swimming pool on the weekend and after work. It worked. At the end of the summer my body was almost as suntanned as it had been in Odessa.

Later, I improvised. To save time and in addition to going to the public swimming pools, I started taking sunbaths on my deck, at the back of our house. I started earlier, in March. It was still cold at that time of the year, but if I lay down under the sun it was warm and comforting, the cold wind blowing some inches above my body.

The sun was my life! It gave my body plenty of vitamin D, the reason I had never been sick in Baltimore. My vitamin D levels were probably 100 ng/ml, or close to it. Having vitamin D levels close to 100 ng/ml closed the gate to diseases or infections.

In San Francisco, the weather was the opposite of that in Baltimore. It was the most torturous weather in the whole world. Many times, the front page headlines in *The San Francisco Chronicle* reported on the brutal and torturous weather. It was always freezing cold, with piecing winds like a thousand daggers piercing my body. Nothing could be saved from the frigid assault, only taking cover inside a car or a building would do.

Sometimes the sun would shine, but I would wear a hat and sunglasses, with my body wrapped in winter clothes. I couldn't find any clothes that would effectively shield me from the cold winds. Even ski jackets could not protect from the wind's assault.

That was why in San Francisco, there were no mosquitoes, as the temperature was never warm enough to hatch their eggs. There were also no air conditioners in homes either, but the heater was on all year around. I had been living in San Francisco for 4 years without sun and vitamin D. The vitamin D that was stored in my body in Baltimore had depleted a long time ago, plus I was older. That was why my immune system broke down and dangerous illnesses infected me.

HOW MEDICAL CARE IN THE USSR AND EUROPE CURED PATIENTS WITH THE SUN

When patients in the Soviet Union became ill, physicians send them to spas. In the USSR and in Russia today, patients were sent to sanatoriums (spas) to be under the sun, to take mud baths, drink mineral water, eat a special diet, and perform aerobic exercises.

To entertain people, in the evening dancing, movies, concerts, and popular lectures occurred. There were lots of spas in the southern part of the country. Patients were sent to spas as sun worshipper for 2–4 weeks to cure their illnesses and get healthier.

After having an operation, patients were often "treated" with the sun. I remember when my best friend had her appendix removed in the hospital. I visited her a few times and saw that immediately after her operation, her bed was wheeled from her room to the balcony, under the sun, so she could recover faster.

Young children were exposed to the sun during the summer. They were sent for the whole summer to summer camps located on the seashore. Summer camps were magical. We started our morning with physical exercises, repeating a motto: "Sun, air, and water all are very good for us." Then we swam or played different sports and games almost all day outside.

As for kindergarten children, during the winter, 2 times per week, the children were put into the sunroom with ultraviolet rays, so their small bodies would get vitamin D and remain healthier during the winter.

Let's consider the following experiment. Sun is life! Don't believe it? Let's take a healthy green plant from outside (the sun) and bring it inside the house and put it into a dark closet. In 6–7 days, diseases will start attacking the plant.

First, the leaves will get red and blue colored spots will appear, then the plant will stop blooming. The leaves will then dry up and fall off. Soon the plant will die. A person's immune system is more complicated than a plant's and requires much more exposure to the sun.

WHAT WAS MY NEXT STEP?
After I gathered all the above information and was 100% sure that only the sun could cure me, I could not wait for the morning to arrive. I called Dr. Morley and told him my discovery in short. He agreed with me and found one lab that was performing a vitamin D test.

At that time, the test was rare and there were hardly any labs that performed the test.[1] I took the blood test, and it showed my vitamin D was virtually zero. Dr. Morley remarked, "You must move immediately to San Diego to be under the sun. Here, in San Francisco, you are going to die."

San Diego was not familiar to me: I had only been there 2 short times as a tourist. I was sick, had no energy, nor any strength to learn about a new city. I decided to go to a place that was more familiar to me. That was Tampa, Florida. I moved there, and spent the first 6 months under the sun,

3–4 hours every day during periods before 10 a.m. and after 3:00 p.m. Then a wonder happened—I recovered! The sun truly was life! It cured me.

DISSEMINATING INFORMATION ABOUT SUN CURE

After my recovery, I was itching to share this important information with the world. I gave my lecture to anyone I met and was willing to listen. When concluding I reminded them that now that they knew the miracle of the sun, they had a personal duty to get rid of their illnesses as the status of their health was now under their control! It was not under the control of anything else, for example, the health care system.

For example: The national news reported the results of a study conducted in New York on children between the ages of 4 and 12. The results showed that children who lived in Manhattan had 2–3 times more incidences of diabetes, asthma, allergies, and other illnesses compared to the children that lived in Brooklyn. Why such a difference? What was the reason?

It was simple. Manhattan had very tall buildings, which shaded the streets and never allowed the sun to shine on the children. Brooklyn was a family neighborhood with single houses, 1–2 stories in height; the sun shined on children all day.

The sun is life and cured all the children from illnesses and diseases in Brooklyn. On internet there are thousands of examples, articles, studies, and research on how the sun cures illnesses.

What about skin cancer or melanoma? Let's use facts and common sense. Melanoma was invented recently in 2005 approximately and is a billion dollar industry. Before 2005, did you hear anything about melanoma? Ask your mother or grandmother, did they know about it? Or have it? Never.

Look at Europeans: they worship the sun. Go to Paris in August. Paris is empty, only tourists are there at that time. All Parisians have headed to the south, to be under the sun all month (they have vacations for 1 month versus Americans 2 weeks).

Search the internet. One can find information about how the majority of melanoma operations in the USA not necessary. Many test results are incorrect and produce the false positives; for example, indicating that a patient has melanoma, when he does not.

Sun protection like SPF creams are very dangerous, as many studies have indicated. SPF cream consists of a dozen chemicals: they react with each other on a person's skin and, as a result of such strong chemistry, can produce melanomas.

In other news headlines like, "Swimmers' Sunscreen Killing off Coral Reefs," even coral reefs are dying from the dangerous SPF cream when sunbathers swim in the water.

□ □ □

THE MORAL OF THE STORY

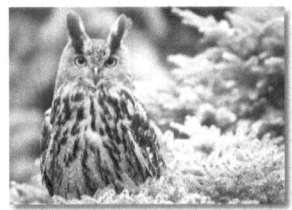

The sun is life; it can cure any illness. The sun is the #1 cure for all illnesses. The internet is full of articles and examples about how the sun has cured many patient illnesses, including cancer. In ancient times, when people relied on common sense and observations of life around them, they worshiped the sun. The sun was a God.

---

[1] For vitamin D a correct test is: 25 — hydroxy vitamin D test. Normal range = 30-100 ng/ml.

SHORT STORY

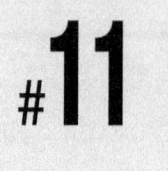

HONEY IS A MEDICINE

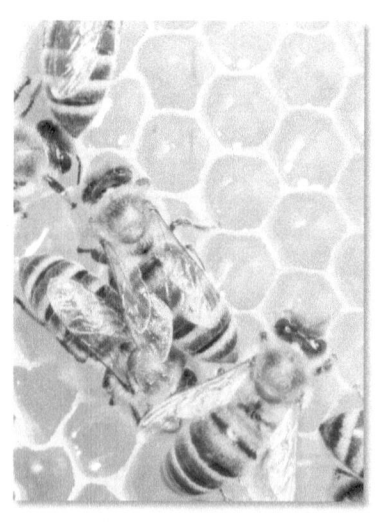
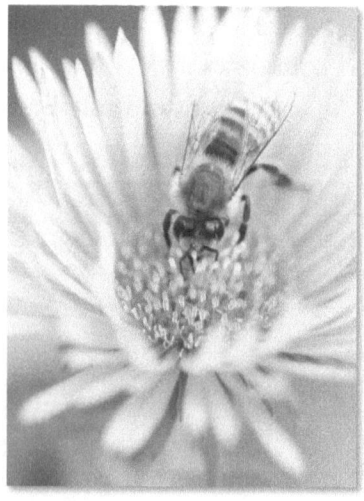

WHAT IS LIFE? WHAT IS HAPPINESS?

□ □ □

ALLERGIES

After living in Maryland, the USA, for several years, my then husband, Chrys, developed a severe summer allergy. It was not an ordinary allergy. Besides coughing, having a stuffy and running nose, and watery and itchy eyes, he had a high fever.

He was miserable and very sick. He could not take any sick leave, as he was a physician, and worked long hours late into the evening, until 10:00 p.m. He tried many allergy medications, but none cured his allergy or were in any way helpful.

His suffering was so bad that we had no choice but to disturb our life and the children's and move to Florida. When we were on vacation in Florida, he had no allergy. With that news, I called my grandmother Anna in Odessa, in the Soviet Union.

HOW TO CURE AN ALLERGY

When I was growing up with my grandparents, they always solved my many problems with very simple solutions. This time was no different. My wise and experienced grandma had a solution. She said, "Give him some honey every morning."

I bought a jar of honey from the supermarket, and so as not to alarm Chrys, quietly put a honey jar in the middle of the kitchen table, next to the grape jam. He liked French breakfasts: toasted bread with cheese and jam, a glass of orange juice, and a cup of coffee. I told him nothing about the honey, as I was afraid that if he knew that the honey was a recipe from grandma to cure his allergy, he would never try the honey.

So, my game started. I was as quiet as a mouse and watched the action. A few days passed, and he kept ignoring the honey jar. Then, curiosity took over him. He tried the honey and liked it. I noticed that he started putting honey on his toast during breakfast.

In less than 3 weeks, his suffering stopped. His allergy was gone and his fever had disappeared for good; he had recovered completely. Sometime later, I told him how my grandma Anna cured his allergy. He made no attempt to disagree with me. No one can disagree with success. He just smiled like a cat that had just swallowed the canary.

For him, the long-awaited relief from his allergy had arrived, and he did not want to jeopardize this by not eating the honey. He continued having it every day, during the fall and winter, and then throughout the year.

Many years later after we were divorced, the children visited him, and brought me news about the honey. Even today, a jar of honey sits prominently in the middle of his kitchen table.

WHAT IS LIFE? WHAT IS HAPPINESS?

Why did the honey cure his severe summer allergy, when numerous medications had no effect on his sufferings? To find an answer, let's use common sense and some observations. Bees, to make honey, fly long distances, often 2–3 miles in radius from their hives, looking for many flowers to pollinate.

And what are the flowers? Flowers are filled with nutrients and vitamins; they are "medicine" and have medicinal powers to cure. In honey, there may be 20–40 different types of flowers, and the bees collect pollen from each of them. Among the many different types of pollen, there were some that helped Chrys to cure his summer allergy.

Today, in less developed countries (over 195 countries), people are curing illnesses and diseases using Nature's remedy. They cannot afford expensive drugs that never cure anything, but are riddled with dangerous side effects. Some of the side effects can even be lethal.

When I was living in Africa, I saw that the Africans were using dry flowers, grasses, leaves, roots, and other organic vegetation to cure illnesses.

Also, I remember when growing up in Odessa, the USSR, we had one neighborhood pharmacy that was serving a surrounding population within a 3–4 kilometer radius. My grandma would send me to this pharmacy to fill up her herbal prescription.

At that time, her prescription was not for a drug. Russian physicians, instead of drugs, very often prescribed a "herbal compound" to patients. The compound was a mixture of vegetation, dry flowers, grass, leaves, and roots.

The pharmacy's glass shelves and cabinets were filled with such natural potions. An aroma from the dried flowers permeated the air. A pharmacist would pick up the herbs "to fill up the prescription" and then like a chief, chop and grind the herbs into a powder and dilute it with some alcohol, glycerite or water, before filling up small bottles with this substance.

Those were the good old days. Today everything has changed. The old pharmacy in Odessa that served the whole neighborhood has gone and been replaced with over a dozen drug stores. They are on every corner of the street selling only expensive pharmaceutical drugs.

Today across the USA, there are many herbal stores that are selling only herbs for different illnesses. Such stores are growing in popularity with the American public.

BUYING HONEY

One important fact about buying honey today. In the 1970s and 1980s, when I started buying honey to cure my then husband's summer allergy, the honey at that time was very close to an organic natural honey. Today, honey has become a commercialized. Companies, to enhance their profits, replaced the natural pollen in the honey with artificial chemicals and preservatives.

Recently, there were news reports about the quality of honey. To conduct the study, the researchers bought many jars of honey from several major stores, drug stores, and other outlets that sold it. A test was conducted to find out how much pollen existed in a jar filled with honey. They found little pollen in the honey in any of the jars they bought and tested except for 2 jars: one was organic honey from Trader Joe's; another was from Whole Foods.

□ □ □

THE MORAL OF THE STORY

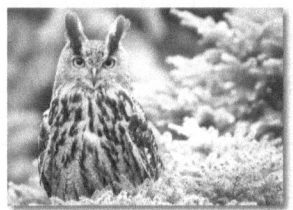

Honey is a natural medicine. It can cure allergy symptoms and other illnesses. For it to act as medicine, the jar of honey you buy must have pollen in it.

In the USA today, pollen in honey has been replaced with artificial substances and preservatives, all designed for profits. Natural honey is relatively expensive when compared to artificial honey.

SHORT STORY

#12

AFRICA: PAST, PRESENT, AND FUTURE

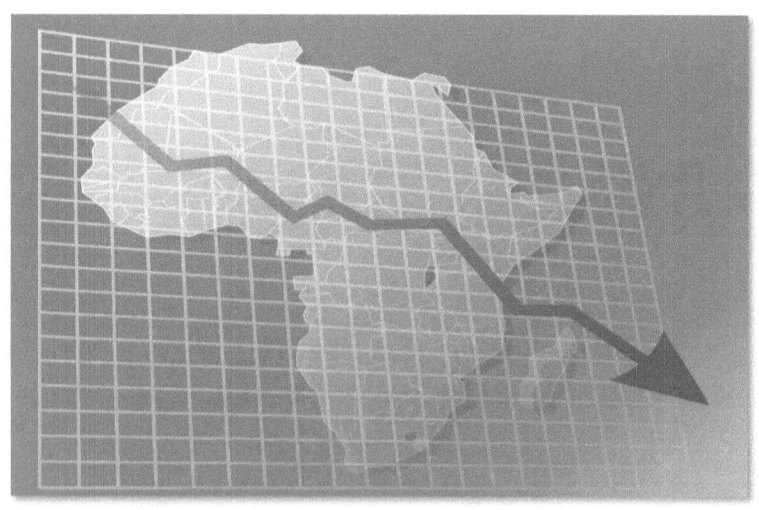

WHAT IS LIFE? WHAT IS HAPPINESS?

□ □ □

In the 1960s, the African continent was boiling. Africa revolted and overthrew its colonial overlords and one by one, 50 or so countries obtained their independence.

This historic event attracted hundreds of thousands of foreign specialists and Peace Corps volunteers who came to Africa to help the new countries build and succeed at their independence.

Foreign economic aid was pouring into Africa. Many countries were competing with each other to show their technical progress and their scale of aid to Africa.

They built superstructures, factories, hospitals, railways, highways, suburbs, and cities across Africa.

At the start of the drive towards independence, Africa had no human resources to run its economies, nor did they have money for economic development. That is why many rich and developed countries came in to help the Africans.

Hundreds of thousands of Africans went to the Soviet Union, China, East Europe, West Europe, and the USA to get a university education, learn new skills, and get trained in military combat and defense.

Towards the end of the 1960s, I was working in Rwanda and Tanzania as a structural engineer and was involved in the African development process.

THE OIL EMBARGO OF 1973–74 DEVASTATED AFRICA AND INTERRUPTED ITS PROGRESS

Suddenly, without any warning, African dreams were interrupted. The world changed and foreign aid to Africa stopped abruptly. What was the trigger? The Oil Embargo of 1973–74. In October 1973, Arab members of OPEC (Organization for Petroleum Exporting Countries) declared an oil embargo on the USA and other West European nations who supported Israel's Yom Kipper War.

The USA and Western Europe were stunned. The embargo stopped their postwar prosperity that was built on cheap energy and cheap raw materials. Overnight, a barrel of oil went from $3.00 to $12.00 per barrel, plus OPEC cut the production of oil. In the USA many gas stations were empty and filling up a vehicle was a challenge. One had to wake up at 5 a.m. and if lucky, could fill up their gas tank.

The embargo also changed the economies of the USA and Western Europe. Western Europe got the shortest end of the stick, as it had no oil resources and relied solely on imports of this scarce commodity.

In 1974, the USA and Western Europe had no other alternative but to oblige OPEC and pay for imported oil at 4 times the pre-embargo cost, leaving their economies acutely strained. And what did the developed countries do? They cut all foreign aid to Africa, resulting in all foreign specialists leaving Africa. Africa was devastated.

WHAT IS LIFE? WHAT IS HAPPINESS?

At that time, in 1973, I was already living in the USA, but keenly watched the changes and effect the Oil Embargo had on Rwanda and Tanzania.

In Tanzania, all development stopped and was frozen, as if some kind of natural disaster had devastated its booming life. Foreign specialists, volunteers, and various missions all left and disappeared. Factories that before were producing goods and equipment for the population broke down from a lack of spare parts and an absence of foreign technicians, who before were running the factories.

Soon, domestic and wild animals started wandering around and the jungles moved in, overtaking factories with bushes and trees.

Cities' superstructures that had been under construction before were now standing idle; only rusty decaying cranes were the reminder that the expectation of ever finishing the construction projects was nil.

Hospitals had no supplies, equipment, or medications, not even aspirin. Crime skyrocketed. Before, during the independence boom, illiteracy among Tanzanians was almost eradicated and armies of villagers moved into big cities for better jobs and opportunities. Now that jobs were gone and the cities could not feed them, they resorted to the one alternative they had—crime.

My friend Natalie, a Russian lawyer who still lives in Dar es Salaam, is highly educated, bright, and very adaptable to any situation. She occupied a very prominent position in the Ministry of Finance and transmitted this information to me on how dramatically life changed in Tanzania.

She tried to build her personal house and in the end gave up. She would buy construction materials, hire guards to guard it day and night, and start construction, but 1–2 months later, all the construction materials would be looted. She would try again, and the looting was repeated months later.

Before its independence in 1964, Tanzania was the poorest country in Africa, with a population of around 10 million.

After independence, it received the highest amount of foreign aid, and as of today, it continue to receive the most foreign aid. The results? Today, or 50 years later, Tanzania still remains the poorest country in Africa. Nothing has changed.

Why can't Tanzania improve the quality of life for its citizens? Because it continues an explosive population growth. No amount of foreign aid can catch up with its population growth from 10 million to 47 million today, an almost 500% increase in 50 years.

The same is true for Rwanda. In 1962, Rwanda's year of independence from colonialism, its total population was 3 million. In 2012, it was 11.5 million, or a 3.8 times increase.

This number is after continuous genocides, the biggest of which occurred in 1994, when almost 1 million Tutsi were massacred.

THE ECONOMIC STATUS OF AFRICA TODAY

Africa's dreams were interrupted the 1st time by the Oil Embargo of 1973–1974, when overnight, the USA, Western Europe, and other countries started paying OPEC $12.00 for a barrel of crude oil instead of $3.00.

They stopped foreign aid to Africa. Later, they resumed the aid and many more countries in the world joined them and, as of today, many countries around the world continue giving aid to Africa.

Foreign aid, as seen from this typical Tanzanian example, has made not even a small dent in improving the quality of life for the average African citizen. Even though Tanzania receives the largest amount of foreign aid in Africa, its poverty remains the same as it was before its independence in 1964. Why? The Tanzanian population exploded from 10 million in the 1960s to 47 million today, an almost 5 fold increase.

The same pattern is true across the African continent. After colonialism in the 1960s, the African continent had 250 million people. Today, or 50 years later, it has exploded to over 1.1 billion, or an increase of 4.4 times, and this unstoppable growth continues upward.

Overpopulation has brought hunger, malnutrition, AIDS, disease, and endless wars between neighboring countries and inside between different cultural and ethnic groups. Today they are fighting for scarce resources to live and survive.

The jungles and wild exotic animals have almost disappeared, the population is moving in taking over the wild life's natural habitat, killing wild animals, reclaiming the jungle, and planting domestic crops for their survival.

Deforestation of jungles has changed the African climate. The climate has become volatile and destructive, with hot temperatures, drought, fires and changes in soil fertility, allowing nothing to grow on it.

The snow-capped view of the Kilimanjaro, a major tourist attraction years ago, today has changed dramatically. The snow has melted from the tallest picks of Kilimanjaro peaks, the wild animals have become extinct, and the thick green jungles that covered the lower mountain elevations are withering into rusty colors.

Fewer exotic safaris are taking place in Kilimanjaro, versus before, when every morning lions' roars woke up tourists.

It is not by accident that Africans, to get some extra land for farming, are moving into the jungles, cutting the trees and bushes, killing wild life in the process.

THE MORAL OF THE STORY

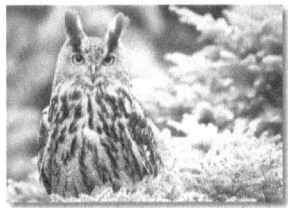

Does Africa have a future? In the 1960s, the African continent overthrew its colonial rulers and became free and independent. This historic event attracted intellectuals and specialist from all over the world who arrived in Africa to help the new countries build their independence and economy.

The foreign aid was pouring into Africa. When the Oil Embargo of 1973–74 quadrupled the oil prices and foreign aid to Africa abruptly stopped, its economic development was derailed and ceased to exist. Later, foreign countries resumed their aid to Africa, but it made no dent in the quality of African lives.

Today, Africa remains as poor as it was before its independence from colonial masters in the 1960s. Why? The African population exploded from 250 million before its independence to 1.1 billion today, or a 440% increase. According to the United

Nation projection by 2050 the population of Africa will double to 2.5 billion.

How much foreign aid does Africa need today to improve the quality of African lives? How many new raw resources are needed to house, dress, and feed 1.1 billion people with the number continue to surge?

How many new continents and land do 1.1 billion people need instead of being cramming into the small African continent today? Sadly, the majority of the world's population is experiencing the same fate and is in no position to alleviate the African misery.

Every complicated problem has a very simple solution. To save Africa's crumbling civilization and to improve the quality of Africans' impoverished lives, Africa should drastically cut its overpopulation explosion. But, that is just my personal opinion.

SHORT STORY

#13

WHAT WAS WORLD WAR II? WHO WON WORLD WAR II? WHAT WAS THE GREAT PATRIOTIC WAR?

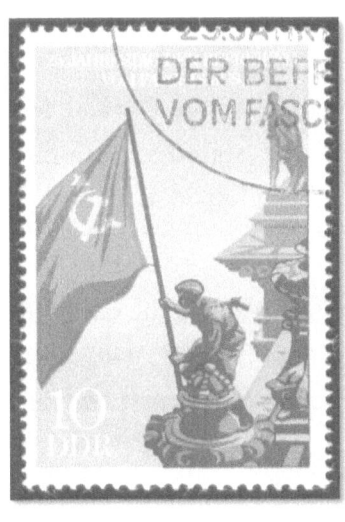
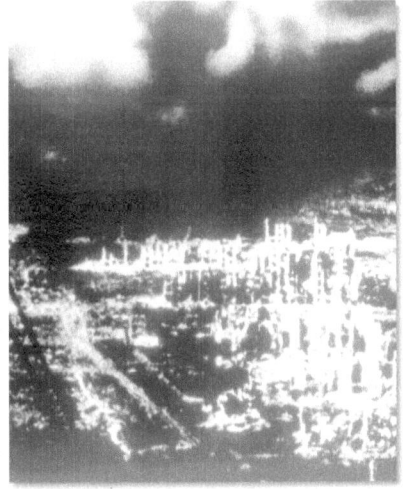

WORLD WAR II, 1941–1945

I was a product of World War II. I was born in the former USSR (the Union of Soviet Socialist Republics, or the Soviet Union), during the war. As a toddler, by shear luck, I survived 3 years of bombings. As a child, I endured the loss of my father and uncles on the Russian battlefields; saw hundreds of deaths; and witnessed devastation, hunger, and disease. I grew up very quickly under the suffering of the war.

One morning, when I was 3 years old, I grew up in just one day. That particular morning, I stepped out from my room onto a balcony and found, to my surprise, that the balcony was covered with dozens of children's books.

Curious, I started to look through some of them. I felt happy: the sun was warm, and the sound of calming classical music was coming from a bell-shaped loudspeaker located on the corner of our street.

The previous night Hitler's Army had reached the outskirts of our city, Voroshilovsk, Donbas, and bombed it all night. One of the bombs hit a nearby children's library, and the explosion showered our apartment building with children's books.

WHAT IS LIFE? WHAT IS HAPPINESS?

Soon, terrifying sirens began warning the population to run for cover, and we could see the German bombers in the sky dropping bombs on our city.

That day, the government of the Soviet Union ordered the mandatory evacuation of all civilians from the city. They transmitted evacuation orders through loudspeakers located on each corner of the city streets.

My father, Peter, and all my uncles had been fighting the Germans on the Russian front for the last 2 years. I was a toddler when my father was mobilized to the war. My brother Victor, mother Lisa, and I all lived with my paternal grandparents, Vasily and Anna.

Under the sound of constant sirens warning civilians of the bombing danger, frightened, in fear among the chaos, and with just a few possessions, we headed to a train station where hundreds of thousands of people were trying to board evacuating trains headed in all directions. Our grandparents did not believe we could survive the war and wanted to die in their native city, Odessa, on the Black Sea. That was why they decided to board the train going south to Odessa.

Odessa was under Hitler's occupation from the beginning of the war. For the first 73 days the Ninth Soviet Army, the Black Sea Fleet, and the 700,000 people of Odessa bravely fought Hitler's 4 attempts to conquer the city at the beginning of the war. During the siege and blockade, Hitler bombed and destroyed Odessa. Near death from wounds and starvation, the civilian population left Odessa.

We arrived in Odessa after several weeks of traveling through bomb attacks and surviving train derailments, but we could not stay there, as the city was now ruined.

There was nothing but danger in the city, so we moved to a village 80 to 90 kilometers from Odessa. This time, we traveled by foot and by horse and carriage from one village to another until we reached our grandparents' former village.

We lived there amid constant battles. The Russians liberated our village, the Germans pushed them back, the Russians attacked again, the Germans retreated, and the front line kept changing back and forth between them.

I saw hundreds of soldier and civilian deaths. After the battles, the Red Cross usually came in to scan the battlefields, check the bodies, look for the living and wounded. We had the biggest house in the village, which it was why our house was always the headquarters of the German or Russian armies. We were squeezed into a corner of the house.

In June 1944, we received a telegram informing us that my father had been killed. "Your son, Peter, was killed, heroically defending Mother Russia." The news devastated my grandparents; they did not want to live.

For days, grandma was crying hysterically, asking God, "What have we done to you? Why did you kill our young

WHAT IS LIFE? WHAT IS HAPPINESS?

son, Peter, whose life was still ahead of him and left us old people to live? You should kill us, not our son." In fear, I would cry, clinging to my grandmother's skirt, scared about what was going to happen to us without our grandparents.

One day my grandparents stopped crying and said, "If we die, how will our little grandchildren survive? We must live for them and take care of them in memory of our son, Peter."

After the war, we moved to ruined Odessa, where hunger and disease had descended on the vulnerable population. The buildings were in ruins. There was no place to live and 2 or 3 families would live crumbled together in a 1-bedroom apartment.

When Germans retreated, they blew up the dam holding the Black Sea back from the city, and the population living in the lower elevation of the city drowned. They blew up the water and sanitary systems, so there was no drinking water and only one kind of food: just bread, a half-kilo (1 pound per person) ration per day. Grandpa would get up by 3:00 a.m. and stand in endless lines to get our rations.

Malnourished and anemic, I started school, where the majority of children in my class did not have fathers—they had all been killed in the war.

During the Great Patriotic War, 1941–1945, that took place for 3 years on Russian soil, 26.6 million Russians were killed—almost all men between the ages of 18 and 50.

After the war, the Soviet government called on Russian women to sacrifice, to rebuild the country, and to save the nation.

Women had to work 2 shifts. During the day they worked in factories and on construction sites, and during the night they entered evening high schools, technical schools and universities to obtain degrees so they could replace the dead soldiers in other jobs.

All the women answered the government's call and sacrificed for the next 20 years until they rebuilt the devastated country. They succeeded beyond imagination: by the 1960s 75% of Russian graduates with bachelor degrees were women.

POLITICAL CLIMATE PRECEDING WORLD WAR II

The USA in the 1930s was in a Great Depression. In 1929, the stock market crashed, followed by high unemployment, soup lines, despair, and destitution. At that time, the USA was an agricultural country with no regular army and no strength. It was a separatist nation and had no influence, as it was a marginal player in international affairs.

The Americans did not want to involve themselves in European or world affairs. But the bombing of Pearl Harbor in December 1941 and World War II drastically changed it.

WHAT IS LIFE? WHAT IS HAPPINESS?

Germany in the 1930s was in a similar situation: high unemployment, weak economy, low morale, and no raw resources. It had relied on the Russian Empire for raw resources since the 19th century.

Hitler's Nazi party came into power in 1933, drumming up military mobilization and raising the morale of the Germans, programming them to believe they were a special Aryan race and were in a downward spiral because of the Jews. It was Fascism or nationalist pursuits over all others people.

Hitler diverted Germans' attention from their impoverishment and economic status, promising a bright future under the Nazi party. They all gladly volunteered to lead them.

Hitler created Nazi Germany and began the suppression of the German Communist party. He portrayed the Communists as Jews in the Soviet Union and in Germany, destroying the great German nation.

The Soviet Union had many Jewish revolutionaries occupying important posts (just to name a few, Leon Trotsky, the Russian War Commissioner, was a Jew. The Russian Commissar for Foreign Affairs, Maxim Litvinov, was also a Jew; and Hitler refused to negotiate with him).

Europe and England, before World War II, were the glorious masters of the universe, bold and arrogant. They established the cradle of capitalism. They were rich and self-sufficient. They ruled over African colonies, India, and the Middle East where they could pump free oil, extract raw resources, and then bring these resources to Europe through the Suez Canal (it opened in 1869, the Suez Canal connected the Mediterranean Sea and the Red Sea through the Gulf of Suez).

The USSR, or the Soviet Union, was a relatively young state and young government with a new socialist system. Before that, it was the 700-year-old Russian Empire which took 1/2 of Asia and 1/3 of Europe under its dominance. The supreme Ruler was an Emperor, or a Russian Tsar. The last Tsar was Nicholas II Romanov.

The Social Democratic Labor Party, led by Vladimir Lenin, staged the Russian Revolution of November 1917, deposed the imperial autocracy, and established a worker and peasant state.

TO PULL OUT OF WORL WAR I, RUSSIA GAVE RUSSIAN TERRITORIES TO GERMANY IN 1918

To pull out of World War I, Russia gave Russian territories to Germany: the Baltic Sea (Latvia, Estonia, and Lithuania) and the Western part of Ukraine, including the city of Lvov, by signing the Brest-Litovsk Treaty in November 1918.

The Russian Revolution of November 1917 had a major impact on World War I (1914–1918) between Europe, Britain, and the Russian Empire against Germany. The majority of the fighting was between the Russians and the Germans. Then the Russian Revolution of November 1917 took place, under the leadership of the Bolshevik party, Vladimir Lenin. It overthrew the Tsarist Regime, and workers and peasants were now in charge of their own country.

Immediately a Civil War broke out between the counter-revolutionary White Army of Tsar Nicholas II and the new pro-revolutionary Red Army of the Bolshevik party (the Majority party).

The founder of the USSR, Vladimir Lenin, saw impossible difficulties for the new socialist state and the Red Army in fighting 3 wars on 3 fronts: World War I, the Revolution, and the Civil War. Lenin postulated that the capitalists, rich manufactures, and industrialists started the war to make money at the expense of the working class who suffered the most.

For this reason, he sought to pull Russia out of World War I by all means possible. He did. Lenin asked Germany to end the war and sign a peace treaty with Russia.

Germany was in a much better situation than the socialist Russia was and agreed to stop the war with the Russians provided that in return, Russia would give them some Russian territory.

Specifically, Germany wanted to have access to the Baltic Sea[1] (Estonia, Latvia, and Lithuania) and Western Ukraine, including the city of Lvov (next to Poland). Lenin had no other alternative but to agree and so he did.

In November 1918, the Bolshevik government signed the Brest-Litovsk Treaty with Germany, pulled out of the war, and accepted those territorial losses.

Once Russia pulled out of World War I, Germany moved their army from the Eastern Front to the Western Front to vanquish the British and Europeans. The British wanted the Russians back in the war, but Lenin was their obstacle. So they sent their agents to assassinate him.

Lenin lived through 2 serious assassination attempts. The 1st was on January 14, 1918; the 2nd was on August 30, 1918. After speaking at a factory in Moscow, Lenin was shot by a British agent Fanya Kaplan, who fired 3 shots and mortally wounded him. She refused to disclose whose agent she was, and the next day she was shot. Lenin had 3 strokes, could not recover from the assassination attempts, and died on January 21, 1924, at age 54.

After Vladimir Lenin's death, Joseph Stalin became the leader of the USSR. Stalin took power and, to industrialize the USSR, established and implemented its first 5-year plan spanning from 1928 to 1932. More 5-year plans followed. By 1939, the Soviet Union had become strong and powerful.

WHAT IS LIFE? WHAT IS HAPPINESS?

It had survived World War I, the November 1917 Revolution, the Civil War, all European, British, and American invasions, as well as sabotages and economic blockades after the Russian Revolution of November 1917.

JOSEPH STALIN DID NOT TRUST EUROPE OR THE BRITISH

After the Russian Revolution of 1917, Europe and Britain were against the Soviet Union's socialism and did not want the young socialist state to survive. They launched sabotages, embargoes, associations of political leaders, and boycotts to cripple the young Soviet state.

The British took advantage of the Russian vulnerability and tried to take some Russian territory. In March 1918, they invaded Murmansk on the Arctic Ocean in the western part of Russia, next to Sweden. In August 1918, the USA invaded Vladivostok, in the Russian Far East, to help the British contingent. The Red Army defeated both Britain and the USA, and expelled them from Russian territories.

After the November Revolution of 1917, in 1922, the 700-year-old Russian Empire was renamed as the USSR (Union of the Soviet Socialist Republics, or the Soviet Union), and later became a powerful nation and a world superpower.

When Europe and Britain failed in getting rid of the Soviet Union this way, they boycotted it economically using embargoes. They stopped trading with the Soviet Union in expectation that the new country, run by inexperienced workers and peasants, could not survive and would perish economically without Europe. They put a wall around the young USSR shutting it off from the outside world.

Later, Western Europe and the Britain arrogantly re-wrote history to their public relations advantage and began calling the USSR the "Iron Curtain." When the facts are that after the 1917 Russian Revolution, it was Europe and Britain who cloaked the "Iron Curtain" around the Soviet Union to suffocate it, economically isolating it from the world.

HITLER INVADED EUROPE IN 1939 AND OCCUPIED IT IN JUST 3 MONTHS

By 1939, Hitler's intoxication with power amplified and he was ready to invade "arrogant Europe and Britain." This time, they had a reason to be arrogant. Europe and Britain were the founders of capitalism and had plenty of wealth and raw resources by exploiting their African colonies, India and the Middle East.

Between 1939–1940, Hitler put the arrogant Europe and Britain to the test: he launched his invasion. France surrendered without firing a single gunshot. The Nazi Army occupied the Netherlands in just one night with a few thousand German parachutists.

Britain was an island and had no raw resources or strategic advantage for Hitler to occupy it. He calculated that to invade Britain, before the USSR, would drain his

WHAT IS LIFE? WHAT IS HAPPINESS?

resources. He reserved to keep Britain under fear, bombing it continually. Hitler occupied the whole of Europe in just 3 months with little resistance.

HITLER'S CLASSIC "TROJAN HORSE" ATTACK STRATEGY TO CATCH THE RUSSIANS OFF GUARD

Joseph Stalin, the leader of the USSR, was suspicious of Hitler's occupation of Europe and demanded an explanation. Hitler reassured him that he had no intention of invading the USSR.

To eliminate Stalin's suspicions, Hitler propositioned him to sign a Non-Aggression Pact between Germany and the USSR. In the Pact, Hitler gave all previous territory that Germany took from Russia after World War I (by the Brest-Litovsk Treaty) back to the USSR.

Before, in the treaty of November 1918, Russia gave Germany the Russian territories: i.e. the Baltic Sea (Latvia, Estonia, and Lithuania) and the Western part of Ukraine, including the city of Lvov.

On August 23, 1939, the Non Aggression Pact between Germany and the USSR was signed. After signing it, Stalin was sure that Hitler had no intention of invading the USSR and was pacified. He stopped all preparation for the war to defend the USSR against Hitler.

Why did Hitler give back Russian territories to the USSR in August 1939? Hitler knew that he could not defeat

Russians in head-to-head war or combat. No one ever had before. He needed to employ deceptions, baits, tricks, and manipulations as an alternative military strategy were he to achieve victory. That strategy was to pacify Stalin—thereby catching Russia off guard and unprepared for an invasion to come.

It was the classic "Trojan Horse" attack strategy. In the Brest-Litovsk Treaty he implemented his Trojan Horse strategy by giving back Russian territories, in exchange for conquering the entire Soviet Union Empire.

Hitler's dream was, the same as that of all previous invaders of Russia: to conquer the richest and the largest country in the world—the USSR, which hold 1/6 of the world's landmass. That was the reason why in the Non-Aggression Pact he gave back the smaller territories to the USSR as bait.

In the 700-year-old history of the Russian Empire, many empires and countries had marched on Russia: Genghis Khan, the Tatars, Turks, Mongols, Japanese, British, Italians, French, and the Germans. The Russians defeated, destroyed, and threw out all of them.

Hitler's top secret plan "Operation Barbarossa" to invade the USSR was strategized for years. In that strategy, Hitler's bait-and-switch tactic served to disarm Stalin's suspicions, allowing Hitler to invade the USSR and catch Stalin surprised and unprepared. Hitler's Trojan Horse strategy worked.

WHAT IS LIFE? WHAT IS HAPPINESS?

ON JUNE 22, 1941, HITLER INVADED THE SOVIET UNION AND WORLD WAR II STARTED

After signing the Non-Aggression Pact in August 1939 and after receiving all the Russian territories back, Joseph Stalin was content and ceased all war preparations against Hitler.

An important Soviet spy, who was a member of Hitler's staff, used radio and Morse code and transmitted his message to Moscow: Hitler's plan "Operation Barbarossa"—the invasion of the Soviet Union. Stalin saw the plan. He did not believe the plan was genuine and dismissed it.

On June 22, 1941, Germany launched Operation Barbarossa and invaded the Soviet Union with 203 divisions and thousands of aircraft and the World War II started.

What was Joseph Stalin doing this day? He was far away from Moscow, on vacation in Sochi, fishing on the Black Sea. When one of his guards brought him the message about Germany's invasion, Stalin was silent and continued fishing for the next 40 minutes.

Stalin returned to Moscow and for the next 4 years lived in the war meeting room located in basement of the Kremlin, where he and his generals designed war strategies and commanded the front. He ate in the same room he slept in and would sleep on the same leather sofa each night. Joseph Stalin was a military genius; without him, the USSR could not win World War II.

BATTLES OF MOSCOW, STALINGRAD, AND BERLIN

In the first weeks of World War II, the German Army and its allies (Italy, Romania and Hungary) marched deep into the Soviet Union unchallenged and unopposed.

In the first 3 weeks, the USSR lost 750,000 soldiers, 10,000 tanks, and 4,000 aircraft that the Germans destroyed on the airfields, as they had no opportunity to take off from the ground. In first 6 months, the USSR suffered 4.3 million casualties, and Germany advanced 1,050 miles inside Russia directly to Moscow, the heart of the USSR.

Hitler figured that once he destroyed Moscow, Russian morale would collapse, and the whole country would fall. By October 1941, the Germans were 50 miles from Moscow. Joseph Stalin did not leave Moscow.

Instead, he took a risk and on November 7, 1941, he staged a military parade in Red Square marking the Twenty First Anniversary of the Soviet Revolution. The parade news reverberated across the nation and boosted the morale of the Russian people.

The civilian population of Moscow organized its own brigades to stop the Germans. The Germans tried but could not get through the Russian defense of Moscow.

In December 1941, the Russian Army counter-attacked and defeated the Germans, but the Russian casualties were staggering. The Battle of Moscow was the 1st single defeat of the Germans; they lost 400,000 men. For the Russians it was a psychological uplift.

The Battle of Stalingrad was Hitler's new strategy. Defeated in Moscow, he changed his war tactics by invading Stalingrad on the Volga River. He was now sure he could defeat Moscow by blockading Stalingrad. Stalingrad was the main blood artery for Moscow's energy, military, and civilian supplies.

By destroying the seaport at Stalingrad (now Volgograd), Hitler hoped to claim Moscow. On August 23, 1942, Germany and its allies started massive bombings that reduced the city to rubble. The Battle of Stalingrad lasted 5 months and was one of the bloodiest battles in the war history. The average life of a Russian soldier in Stalingrad's battle was 24 hours.

On February 2, 1943, the Soviet Army defeated the Germans and their allied armies in Stalingrad. And 2 major German generals, Van Paulus and Schmidt, with another 22 generals and what was left of their armies, surrendered. Stalingrad was a turning point in World War II. The Russian casualty count was over 1.1 million; for the Germans and its allies it was 850,000. The population of Stalingrad fell from 850,000 habitants before the war to 1,500 after the war.

In exchange for his captured general Von Paulus, Hitler proposed an even exchange to Joseph Stalin, through the

Red Cross: he wanted to exchange Von Paulus for Stalin's eldest son, Yakov.

Yakov was a lieutenant in the Soviet Army and was captured by the Germans on July 16, 1941, during the battle of Smolensk, during the initial stages of the German invasion of the Soviet Union. Stalin replied, "I could not exchange a soldier for a general." The Germans shot Yakov on April 14, 1943.

The West characterized this event, "Joseph Stalin was very cruel: he did not even want to save his own son." Not the Russians—they interpreted Stalin's answer as that of a great leader. Many millions of Russian men were killed by Hitler's Army. Why should Stalin's son Yakov be different and privileged? If Stalin had exchanged Von Paulus for his son, the Russian people would have lost respect for him as their leader.

After Stalingrad victory, the war turned, and the Soviet Red Army began pushing the Germans back. By June 1944, the Soviet Army had liberated all the USSR territory and continued pursuing the Germans back to Berlin, liberating along the way all European countries that Hitler had occupied in just 3 months, between 1939 and 1940.

Now an alliance, the USA and Britain—seeing that the USSR had defeated Hitler and that the Soviet Army had liberated Europe, became afraid of the USSR, imagining that it could annex all of Europe under their socialist umbrella.

They decided to open their second front, 3 years later, on June 1944, called the Normandy landing where 10,000 Allied soldiers were killed. (The World War II started on June 22, 1941—when Hitler invaded the Soviet Union.)

In the Battle of Berlin, the major Hitler stronghold, the USA and Britain did not participate with the Soviet Red Army, as they were not sure of their strength. The Battle of Berlin was again a Russian affair; it lasted from April 20, 1945, to May 2, 1945. The Russian general-genius Georgy Zhukov was the commander; 81,116 Soviet soldiers were killed in this battle, and 280,251 were wounded.

General Zhukov, as the legend goes, addressed his Soviet Army immediately after the battle: "My dear Comrades, you saw your Mother Russia get destroyed and leveled; many millions of Russians were killed, but do not retaliate against the Germans.

"You are the victor; you won the war and defeated Fascism. Remember who you are: you are the great, stoic, and proud people who saved the world from Fascism. Carry your dignity and honor with pride and show mercy to your enemy." After the battle, the Soviet Red Army opened soup kitchens to feed Germans, and for that the Berlin population was grateful to them.

WHY DID THE USA AND BRITAIN NOT OPEN THE SECOND FRONT FOR 3 YEARS?

THEY ONLY OPENED WHEN THE SOVIET ARMY WAS ALREADY MARCHING ON BERLIN

During World War II, 1941–1945, to stop the Russian bleeding and take some of the heat away from the Russian Red Army, Joseph Stalin continuously asked the USA and Britain to open up the second front against Germany.

The American President Roosevelt and the British Prime Minister Churchill refused, stating that they were too weak to fight the Germans. They opened their second front, 3 years later, on June 1944 with the D-day invasion of Normandy, after the Russians liberated the USSR and Europe and were marching on Berlin.

At the end of World War II, there were big sufferers and big winners. The biggest sufferer was the USSR. The biggest winner was the USA, as described below.

I) THE BIGGEST SUFFERER IN WORLD WAR II WAS THE USSR

In recent history, Russia saved the whole Europe in 1812, by defeating Napoleon in Moscow, after he had conquered all of Europe. The second time the USSR saved Europe was in 1941–1945 when it defeated Hitler in World War II at huge national sacrifice.

The USSR won the war, but at what cost? During the 4 years of World War II, it raged for 3 years on Russian

WHAT IS LIFE? WHAT IS HAPPINESS?

soil, where 26.6 million Russians were killed, almost all men between the ages of 18 and 50. They gave their lives for their Mother Russia and for future generations. And those lucky ones who survived and came back from the front were gravely injured, with missing arms, legs, or eyes, many did not live for long.

The entire country lay in ruins. It was without superstructures, housing, schools, factories, water systems, sanitary systems, and electricity—all had been destroyed and leveled. After the war, hunger and disease descended on the decimated population. Only women, children and old men were left to rebuild the ravaged country.

The war produced many millions of widows with small children. Millions of mothers lost their sons. Many millions of young would-be brides never got married, forgoing a family and children because their future grooms were killed in the war. And 15 million children were orphaned, many of whom were semi wild, living on the streets for 4 years or in ruined buildings and scavenging for food and shelter to survive.

The USSR government faced challenges of epic proportions. How could it stop the hunger and disease? How could it rebuild the country and save the nation? The Soviet government found the solution—Russian women.

They called on Russian women to save the nation and rebuild the destroyed country; they asked them to make huge personal sacrifices so the country would survive and the Russian nation would live. After the war, the USSR's technological clock was turned back decades as the country was leveled and in ruins. It took decades to rebuild what was lost.

The Soviet government asked Russian women to work 2 shifts every day, 16 hours a day. They worked on construction sites rebuilding plants, schools, roads, and buildings, and they worked in factories producing goods for the population and arms and supplies for the army.

Then, in the evening, women were to enter schools, universities, and technical schools to become engineers, teachers, physicians, economists, and technicians. Women needed to receive this education in order to replaced the men who had been killed.

All of the Russian women answered the government's call. They sacrificed, and in 15 to 20 years, they rebuilt the country. Millions of women graduated with bachelor's and technical degrees in engineering, science, education, medicine, economics, accounting, and many technical specialties.

Women sacrificed yet succeeded beyond imagination. Less than 1 generation later, Russian women outperformed their men. Every year, 75% of Russian women graduated from universities. As for teachers and physicians, more than 90% were women.

The Russians won World War II at a huge cost. That is why in the Soviet history books, the war's correct name is The Great Patriotic War, or, the Patriotic War of the Russian people against Fascism to save civilization.

The West and the USA shamelessly rewrote the war's history, renaming the Russian Great Patriotic War as World War II. According to them, the USA and Britain won World War II and saved the world from Fascism, not the USSR.

II) THE BIGGEST WINNER IN WORLD WAR II WAS THE USA.
IT CHANGED THE COUNTRY FROM BEING A BACKWARD AGRICULTURAL AND SEPARATIST COUNTRY INTO A WORLD SUPERPOWER

As the historical facts show, World War II was a blessing for the USA. It saved the USA from unemployment, and soup lines of the Great Depression of the 1930s. World War II gave jobs to nearly all Americans and drew the isolationist USA into international affairs.

After the war, hundreds of thousands of Germans, afraid of Russian reprisal, and many European engineers and scientists escaping war-devastated Europe, came to the USA, thus creating the military industry and space program, thereby transforming the USA into a world superpower.

For the second time the Russians had saved Europe and Britain. The Russians lost 26.6 million people during the war, and the country was leveled and destroyed. There were 405,399 American military deaths in World War II and 382,700 British deaths.

While growing up in the Soviet Union, at school I learned from history books that the war of 1941 to 1945 was a Great Patriotic War, in which the Russians defeated Hitler and saved Mother Russia, Europe, the world and civilization from Fascism.

When I went to Africa and then to the USA, I was surprised to learn that history had been rewritten. The Russian Great Patriotic War was renamed into the Second World War, or World War II, and the Americans and British had won the war—the Russians were just allies.

What was the gratitude shown by the West and the USA for the Russian sacrifices? How did Europe, Britain, and the USA show how grateful and thankful they were to the USSR for making epic sacrifices, fighting on their soil, winning the war at the expense of 26.6 million Russian lives, dealing with a ruined country, and saving Europe, Britain and the USA from Fascism?

Instead of thanking the Russians for saving them from Hitler, the capitalist powers launched a Cold War aggression. Beginning in 1946, the USA, Britain and Western Europe manufactured the Cold War doctrine against the postwar USSR, sabotaging the Russian post war recovery.

WHAT IS LIFE? WHAT IS HAPPINESS?

They are continue it as of today against Russia—their traditional opponents of capitalist power. Talk is cheap and can be deceiving; but not facts—facts are the truth. Look at the facts and find out who won World War II? The Russians? Or, the Americans and British?

The doctrine of capitalist power is hostility and aggression to another country to start disturbance and war. This is so rich capitalists, such as the military industry, multinationals, banks, and private contractors, can enrich themselves from the war at the expense of the working class, who are made to suffer the most.

History repeats itself today. As this story is being written, the USA, Britain, and Western Europe are doing the same to Russia again. In February 2014, they facilitated a coup in Kiev, Ukraine, where the USA spent $9 billion to overthrow the democratically elected Ukrainian government with their mercenaries in order to install their puppet.

Why? You see, Ukraine is the country closest to Russia culturally and ethnically. Yet, with Ukraine bordering Europe, it has proven to be an irresistible target for the destabilization by the West, leading the destabilization of Russia herself.

The West and USA leaders do not like President Vladimir Putin—all because he is not an American puppet, as leaders of Europe and Britain are. Instead, Putin is a nationalistic and patriotic leader; he does what is the best for Russia and the Russian people, and not what is best for the USA.

The USA bombs and invades any country on faraway continents any time when they cannot control or do not like their leaders. Vietnam, Korea, Yugoslavia, Granada, Iraq, Afghanistan, Libya, and Syria are just a few examples.

Today it is Ukraine, even though 85% of Americans don't have any idea where Ukraine is located. Nevertheless Western powers do not care about Ukraine's prosperity, but instead use it like a pawn in an international chess match against Russia. This is traditional hostility of a capitalist power.

By comparison, if Russia condoned a coup d'état in Mexico such that Mexico could be managed, even controlled by Russia, how would the American people feel?

THE MORAL OF THE STORY

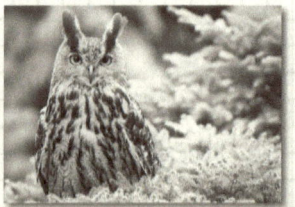

What was World War II? Who won World War II? The Russians, or the USA and the British? Let's not believe historical revisionism but instead believe in the truth. Look at the facts and make your own conclusions and judgments. Propaganda is cheap

WHAT IS LIFE? WHAT IS HAPPINESS?

and purposely deceitful, but the facts are not. Facts are the truth.

Indisputable facts from World War II indicate that Hitler invaded and occupied the whole of Europe in just 3 months without any resistance. Then, on June 22, 1941, Hitler invaded the Soviet Union and the World War II started.

Unexpected and unprepared, the Russians suffered heavy causalities but fought valiantly and defeated Hitler. By June 1944, the Soviet Army liberated the Soviet Union and started liberating Europe as it marched to Berlin.

Where were the Americans and the British all this time? They did not enter World War II immediately. Why? For 3 years Joseph Stalin asked them to enter the war and stop the Russian bleeding. President Franklin D. Roosevelt and Prime Minister Winston Churchill replied: "We are too weak to fight Hitler."

Only 3 years later, in June 1944, seeing that the Soviet Army was marching to Berlin, they feared that Joseph Stalin would occupy the whole of Europe. That is when they opened the second front and launched the Normandy landing.

World War II was fought on Soviet soil for 3 years. The entire country was destroyed and leveled, and 26.6 million Russians were killed, almost all men between the age of 18 to 50. Millions of Russian widows were left with small children; millions of mothers lost their sons; and millions of young, future brides never were able to marry or raise families because their grooms-to-be were killed. And 15 million orphans were left behind, many of them semi wild, living during the war on the streets and in ruined buildings, fending to stay alive.

That was the Soviet Union's Great Patriotic War, as it was correctly called in history books. Later, the USA and Britain bluntly rewrote the war's history. They renamed Russian's Great Patriotic War as World War II, and the victors were the USA and Britain, with minor involvement from the Soviet Union.

Growing up in the Soviet Union, I started the 1st grade after the war. In my class there were only 6 children with fathers, the rest of us had no fathers—all were killed. I always kept dreaming about what life could have been like if I had a father. In school, we learned from history books that the war of 1941 to 1945 was the Great Patriotic War of the Soviet Union.

The Russians defeated Hitler and saved Mother Russia, Europe, the world and mankind from Fascism. Then, when I went to Africa and then came to the USA, I was surprised that history has been rewritten.

The total number of deaths in World War II were: 26.6 million Russians deaths, 405,399 American military deaths, and 382,700 British deaths. Britain and the USA contributed the least to the war. Those are the facts; they do not lie.

The Soviet Union won World War II and saved the world and civilization from the Fascism in the Great Patriotic War.

---

[1] Population of Baltic Sea republics: Estonia = 1.0 million in 1940, 1.6 mil. in 1991, 1.3 mil. in 2013. Latvia = 1.9 million in 1940, 2.6 mil in 1991, 2.0 mil in 2013.
Lithuania = 2.6 million in 1940, 3.7 mil in 1991, 3.0 mil in 2013. After the Soviet Union disintegrated in 1991, the population of those Baltic Sea republics decreased by 20%.

SHORT STORY #14

COWARDS. OR, BLOOD IS THICKER THAN WATER

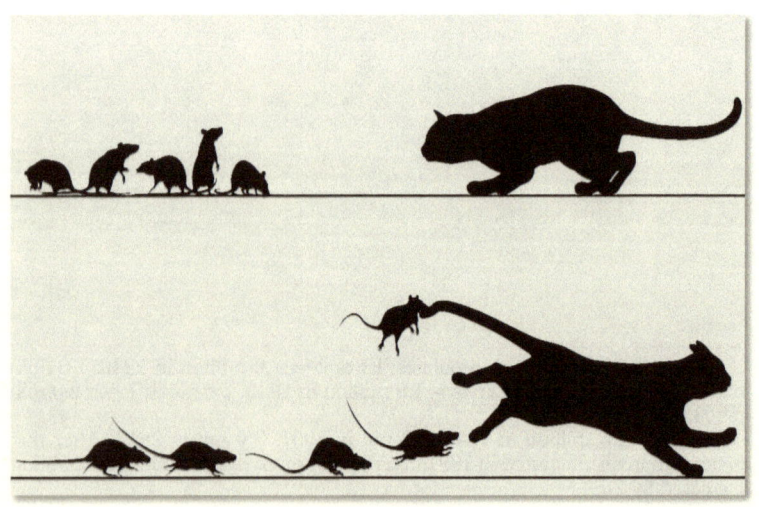

WHAT IS LIFE? WHAT IS HAPPINESS?

□ □ □

"The blood is thicker than water."
Grandpa Vasily

"Do not be a coward, instead defend yourself." My grandpa Vasily was teaching me new traits of character. "Stand up and defend yourself if you can, your brother, family, friends, school, society, and the country," he continued.

He meant stand behind them, express your opinion orally (if appropriate)—not fight physically with your fists. To my young and inexperienced mind, this law of life was difficult to comprehend. It was not clear to me what my grandpa wanted to install in me. As usual, he gave me a visual example to better comprehend his law of life.

"You see," grandpa reasoned, "when during the war Germans captured Russian soldiers, they treated them with some sort of dignity. They did not shoot them immediately; instead, they put them into the prisoners of war camps." He stopped for a minute and kept silent, waiting for me to have some time to differentiate among his 2 analogies.

Then, he introduced a 2nd and opposite analogy. "But, when a Russian coward soldier defected to the Germans by crossing the frontline, the German treated him with disgust. The 1st thing they did was question him to get strategic information on the movement of Russian troops, their defense strategy, and their next actions.

"After they squeezed from the coward all the information he had, or the Germans needed, they stopped and remunerated the coward. How do you think they remunerated the coward who sold Russian soldiers' lives to Germans?

"Immediately, they marched him outside and shot him. Why? Very simple, if this coward-defector could easily sell to his enemy his country, his comrade soldiers, parents, relatives, friends with whom he speaks the same language, went to the same school, and lived in the same community, then what is going to prevent this coward defector from selling Germans—the enemy of his country?" grandpa asked.

He summarized it in one short sentence, "Blood is thicker than water."

I had no answer, but I knew that grandpa was not waiting for my answer. He, as usual, was giving me new information to develop my young character, or just plant a seed into my mind, so he thought.

When grandpa attempted to teach me some traits of character, I was not a very good pupil. If only he knew. I did not dare to interrupt him or show any disrespect. On the surface, my body did not move, and I made no disagreements with him, but my 2 ears were divided—1 tried to focus on grandpa and the other was listening for outside activities. My friends in the courtyard of our apartments already were out playing games and jumping rope.

WHAT IS LIFE? WHAT IS HAPPINESS?

Many years passed and this grandpa's lecture was forgotten or lost in a maze of information stored in my mind. When I matured into an adult, astonishingly, my grandpa's law of life from his wisdom about the cowards and "blood is thicker than water" surfaced. Being an adult, I was flooded with everyday challenges to analyze and had to make decisions about events and problems. Some examples are below.

THE DAUGHTER OF THE LEADER OF THE SOVIET UNION DEFECTED TO THE USA

When I arrived in the USA via Africa, here a big international news extravaganza was going on. The daughter of the Soviet Union leader, Joseph Stalin, defected to the West. She was Svetlana Stalina, or Svetlana Alliluyeva (her mother's maiden name). [1]

In 1967, she brought to India the ashes of her Indian husband; she was 42 years old, 3 times married, and left behind her 2 children. She had college degrees in history and in the English language.

In India, she went to the USA embassy asking for political asylum. The USA refused and a CIA agent escorted her to live in Switzerland. Finally, President Lyndon B Johnson agreed to admit her on humanitarian grounds, but wanted to keep it low-key in the news. In a New York airport, she denounced the Soviet Union regime.

Soon, she married for the 4th time, this time to an American, had a daughter and after 2 years of marriage was divorced for the 4th time. Curiously, I was watching news about her and was puzzled why the USA initially refused to give her political asylum.

Why didn't they use such a rare propaganda opportunity during the Cold War against the Soviet Union? Capitalism must be superior to socialism; she was a black eye to socialism, where even the daughter of the president, who had all privileges, could not live there. There were streaming news about her 24/7 across the world.

Soon I learned why. The answer came from my grandpa's lecture that I had listened to with only 1 ear many years ago during my childhood. Cowards who defected from their own countries were looked upon by their enemies not with trust, but disgust. Even though Svetlana Stalina's defection was a billion-dollar piece of propaganda that dropped into Americans' laps for free, deep inside, Americans were repulsed.

How would they have felt if a daughter of then President Lyndon Johnson defected to the Soviet Union, their enemy? Americans feelings of disgust overpowered the free propaganda. To them she was a crazy woman and unstable.

The American public was straightforward—a classic expression was: "I would not trust her [Svetlana Alliluyeva] to even wash dishes in the soldiers canteen."

Svetlana wrote her 2 memoirs, one was "Only One Year" and a publisher bought her memoirs for $2 million, thinking that he could make several million dollars from her books. The publisher's gamble never materialized—not many copies of her memoirs were sold to recuperate the money paid to her.

Later, impoverished and unstable Svetlana kept bouncing between many countries, trying different lifestyles and religions.[2] In 1984, she went back to Moscow where she declared that she was "a pet of CIA" and she "had not known one single day of freedom in the USA."

In 1986, she was back in the USA. By the 1990s, she settled in a shabby part of London for the elderly with mental problems, then back to the USA. She died in Wisconsin in 2011 at the age of 85. Was she an American hero or an unstable and spoiled brat who, as a defector, selfishly wanted to bring some attention to herself?

A SOVIET PILOT STOLE THE MOST ADVANCED MILITARY JET, MIG-25, AND FLEW IT TO JAPAN

Again, almost 10 years later, in 1976, the same repulsion was shown by the USA to another Russian defector, Viktor Belenko. He flew a MIC 25 "Foxbat," a military jet fighter, to Japan. There was a promise from the USA of $100,000 given to anyone who defected to the West bringing with him this fighter plane.

The MIG-25 was a very advanced Soviet military aircraft, a top secret warplane, and its loss caused a lot of damage to the Soviet Union Air Force; it was a windfall to the

Western military. The USA disassembled the MIG-25 and it revealed many secrets and surprises.

After the defector was interrogated and debriefed by the CIA, FBI, and other interested agencies, he was free to go. "To go where?" the defector asked. "Anywhere you want," was the answer. The MIG defector saga was published in *Reader's Digest* magazine and on the front pages of many newspapers. I remembered reading that after the Americans finished interrogating him, he was of no more use to them. They unceremoniously threw him to the street.

The defector, without a country or job, started driving to Washington, D.C. Even he had no more use for the Americans; they did not trust him and considered him unstable. They followed him to see where he was going. When they recognized he was going to the Soviet Union Embassy to re-defect back, they apprehended him.

In 1980, or 4 years after his defection, the Congress in the end granted him citizenship, signed into law by President Jimmy Carter.[3] In the Soviet Union, he was married and had a son who was 4 years old when Viktor Belenko defected.

Soon, he married an American teacher, without divorcing his Russian wife. They had 2 children and 2 years later they were divorced.

He kept giving "lectures" about his life in the Soviet Union across the USA, telling his audience what they wanted to

WHAT IS LIFE? WHAT IS HAPPINESS?

hear: in the Soviet Union they had no canned food; in the USA he ate canned food for the 1st time in his life. He said it was delicious and especially when he learned it was cat food.

He said that in San Francisco, homeless men in the Tenderloin District lived better than Russians; and many more anecdotes. His 2 children were never with him, and he never mentioned to his new friends that he had 2 children here in the USA. He drank hard liquor and laughed hard ("laughing all the way to the bank").

From the mid-1990s, he disappeared from the radar. Was he an American hero or a selfish coward defector who would do and say anything for money?

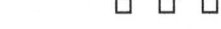

□ □ □

THE MORAL OF THE STORY

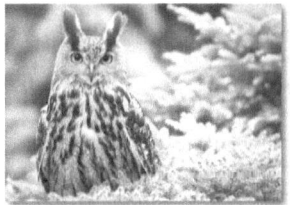

Do not be a coward. Blood is thicker than water. Defectors are not heroes; they are selfish unstable cowards.

A coward or a hero? Svetlana Alliluyeva, Joseph Stalin's daughter, was a privileged spoiled brat. In 1967, she defected to the USA, blaming her defection on her father (who died in 1953) and on a lack of freedom in the Soviet Union. She was 42 years old, already 3 times married, and left her 2 children behind. Was she an American hero or an unstable and selfish coward defector who, to bring attention to herself, defected to the USA?

A coward or a hero? Viktor Belenko, another Soviet defector, in 1976 stole the Soviet Union's top secret MIG-25 warplane and flew it to Japan. The USA wanted to get the MIG-25 fighter technology that flew faster and higher than any fighter to date and promised to give $100,000 to anyone who would bring this plane to the West. Viktor Belenko did.

He blamed his defection on "bad living conditions" in the Soviet Union and the fact that, before his defection, his wife Lyudmila demanded a divorce and planned to take their 4-year old son from him.

Then, in the USA, he got married, had 2 children, and after 2 years was divorced. Now a free man, he traveled across the USA giving his anecdote-filled "lectures" to anyone willing to listen and pay for it, and was "laughing all the way to the bank."

Here, he never mentioned his 2 small children to anyone he drank with, or when traveling across the USA. Was he a hero, or a selfish coward who would do anything for money?

There are many heroes among us and around us. One group is the American soldiers who volunteered to fight in the wars in Iraq and Afghanistan. Many of them died and many returned home wounded. They gave their lives fighting for their country without asking for anything in return.

They put their country, nation and families above their selfish, personal wants. They, the war veterans, are the real Americans heroes! Not the Russian defectors Svetlana Stalina and Viktor Belenko. Other heroes are the 26.6 million Russians who were killed during the Second World War. They gave their lives for their Mother Russia and saved the world from Fascism.

The majority of people are not very keen to any defector. The reasoning is that a defector has sold his family, children, mother, father, brother, his relatives, teachers and friends, all people who brought him up, fed him, cared for him, educated him, and gave jobs to him—people whom he owes everything for his existence.

He has an obligation to give them back something. He was a labor of love of many other people who invested their energy, time, and money in him during the most crucial part of his life: baby, toddler, young child, teen, young adult. Who fed him, cared for him and educated him?

How the defector could not sell out at the first opportunity new strangers in a new country? These strangers that did nothing for him, and he had no obligation to do something great for them.

Some people are just cowards who do not want to grow up and take any responsibility for themselves and their actions. Some TV shows are full of those people. People who reveal on TV their problems of using drugs, conducting criminal activities, violence, jail terms, DUI police arrests, marital infidelities to name just a few.

They always have an excuse for their failures or misdeeds. They never blame themselves; instead they always blame other people close to them: their family or friends, government, IRS and the like.

Never mind that they are already adults and stopped living at home a long time ago. And for many years of adulthood had the opportunity to better themselves and achieve anything they want without parents interference and command. Instead they drifted, wasted their time and when someone pressed them why they accomplished nothing, or misbehaved, they never held themselves accountable and blamed others for their failures and loses. They are weak, selfish cowards versus being selfless people.

---

[1] bbc.co.uk on March 9, 1967 "1967: Stalin's daughter defected to the West."
[2] New York Times "Lana Peters, Stalin's Daughter, Dies at 85," November 28, 2011 by Douglas Martin.
[3] en.wikipedia.org

SHORT STORY

#15

NO MONEY, NO FUNNY.
OR, FROM RENTERS TO HOMEOWNERS

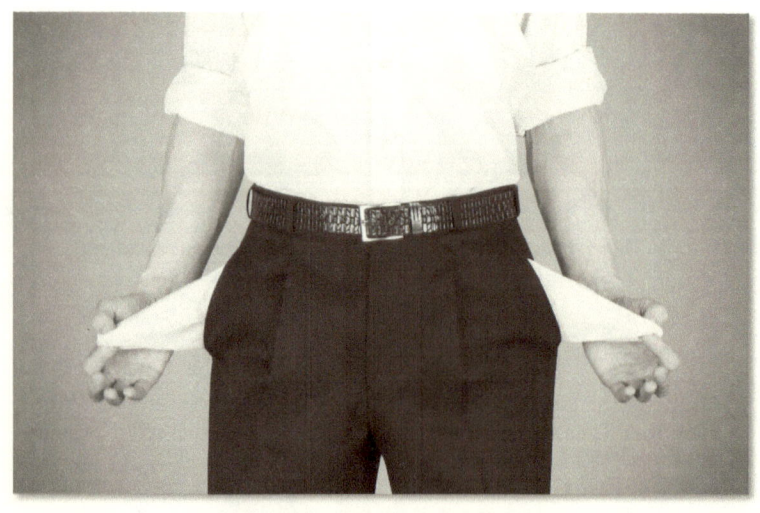

WHAT IS LIFE? WHAT IS HAPPINESS?

□ □ □

A young man named Bob, a new college student was, for the 1st time in his life, far away from home and he had no idea how to plan his everyday spending. Soon he was in trouble; he quickly ran out of money. He knew only one source of money, his parents, and sent the following message to his father:

No money,
No funny,
Sonny.

His father soon replied:

How sad,
How bad,
Dad.

This funny story was in one of my self-teaching English books. Chrys, seeing how effortlessly I studied English using Russian books that were extremely difficult, bought me 4 self-teaching English books, from the beginners stage to the advanced. The books were very easy to read, they used pictures, cartoons, and funny stories to teach students English.

FROM APARTMENT RENTERS TO HOMEOWNERS

When we arrived in the USA in the 1970s and were renting an apartment, we saved tons of money and did not know what to do with the money until we bought a house. Quickly, like in a furnace, our savings went up in smoke.

Our rented 2 bedroom apartment was located in a new apartment complex in Ellicott City, Maryland. The monthly rent was $180, which was just 50% of my 1 week salary as an engineer. The apartment complex had a swimming pool, a small neighborhood store, and a dentist's office; there was also a car wash facility and many huge grassy open spaces.

Moreover, the apartments were located next to a forest. The schools were excellent and there wasn't any crime. Thus there was no need for the children to have baby sitters. Instead, they had latch keys to get in and out of their apartments, and all the children played outside. If by accident they were locked out, they would go to the rental office where employees would gladly help them and open their apartments.

Then one day Chrys came home and announced that this coming Sunday we were going to look at buying a house. He had already been to a real estate agent, and her agency was conveniently located next to his office. This was not news to me because for some time my peers in my office had been encouraging me to buy a house. They wondered why we had not bought one yet, when they had all bought houses already.

From the beginning I was not very eager to buy a house. I grew up in the big, beautiful, metropolitan city of Odessa

WHAT IS LIFE? WHAT IS HAPPINESS?

on the Black Sea, where all the buildings were made up of apartments and life was outside, not inside. School, work, living, and entertainment all took place in the city and I usually came home after midnight just to sleep.

So, on Sunday, the real estate agent drove us around to show us many of the houses for sale. In the end, we found one we liked, bought it, and moved in.

Our apartment rent was $180 per month and the utility bills were very low, totaling a maximum of $50 per month, which was nothing close to our homeowner expenses in the new house. These are what our expenses were in our new house: during the 1st month, we hired a farmer to convert our 2 acres of farmland into a grassy area and paid him $10,000 (today $50,000); then 1 year later, our cathedral ceiling roof started leaking and to repair it, we paid $15,000.

In our ignorance, we did not know that it was the builder who should have repaired and paid for our roof. Our mortgage was $780 per month, with $5,000 per year property tax, and our utility bills were enormous. During the summer, to cool our glass cathedral ceiling house, our electric bill was over $700 each month, and during the winter, our heating bill was $500 per month. The fees for a membership at the neighborhood swimming pool were $600 per summer. This did not include the many thousands of dollars we paid for inside and outside furniture and for wall papering all the rooms.

Plus, we hired 2 contractors at a cost of $500 each to cut the grass during the summer and remove the snow during the winter from our 300 foot long driveway. We also bought new shrubs, planted many new trees and flowers, and bought wood for the fireplace, any many more.

In short, our apartment expenses were $230 per month and as a result, we kept accumulating a lot of money and did not know what to do with it. Then we bought the house and before we knew it, like in a furnace, our money went up in flames.

In total, our house expenses went up to $3,000 per month. We also spent a lot of our time and energy on the house to keep it up and pay for maintenance costs. If we had continued living in an apartment, every 10 years we would have saved over $300,000, or over $700,000 in 20 years by the time we sold our house.

ACCUMULATING STUFF TO PASS THE TIME IS A LOST LIFETIME

After we bought the house and moved in, we started accumulating stuff. When the weekends arrived, what was there to do in the house or tranquil rural neighborhood?

The only recreation was going to the shopping malls, where one went shopping to buy things and accumulate stuff to fill a nostalgic void for entertainment and a social life. About 15 years later, when every space in the house and the garage was now filled up, this condition was brought to my attention—by accident.

WHAT IS LIFE? WHAT IS HAPPINESS?

One morning I was backing out of the garage in my brand new Audi which usually took a lot of skill since the garage was perched on the edge of a hill. Our garage was filled up with numerous boxes and bookcases.

This time, my car bumped into one of those bookcases and an avalanche of stuff crashed down on my car and damaged it. That was a tipping point that made me angry with myself.

Steaming all day and calling to make arrangements for car repairs and a rental car, I could not wait to get back home and start a major project which was to get rid of all the accumulated stuff and clear out my life. I decided that everything that was not used in the last 12 months must go to the Salvation Army, or Goodwill, including expensive clothes with tags still on them and unpacked bags and boxes.

For the next week, inch by inch, we cleaned the house and brought all the stuff into the game room. I gave all of it to the Salvation Army, and then claimed $80,000 on my tax returns which was the market value for the stuff.

The IRS audited me, but I brought all the receipts from the upscale stores and after 20–30 minutes, they accepted my tax deductions, and closed the audit. I was equating accumulated stuff with happiness, but I really lived an empty life by buying things to fill the void, and using malls for entertainment on weekends.

WRAPPED IN DEBT LIKE IN SILK ROBES

"Wrapped in debt like in silk robes" is a wise Russian saying telling people not to wrap themselves up in debt as if they were wearing silk robes. But, people do just that—get buried in debt.

After 29 years of marriage, I filed for divorce and later was hit with huge legal bills. At the same time, I did not lower my spending, but continued the same level of spending on useless stuff and soon I was in trouble. I was wrapped up in debt as if I was wearing silk robes. It was only after this I learned my lesson and stopped going to the mall to fill up my emptiness with "stuff."

Today Americans, as per the Federal Reserve, have $17 trillion in household debts and over $1.1 trillion in student loan debts.

During the "subprime mortgage" scam from 2000–2008, Americans went on a borrowing spree and took home an equity line of credit at high interest rates thinking that home values would continue going up, as if the sky was the limit. Then in September 2008, the economy collapsed and they were left holding on to huge debts.

Surveys indicated that they spent all of their home equity loans on vacations, buying new cars, and installing new granite kitchen countertops. The average American has the following debts: credit card debt $16,000; student loan debt $34,000; and the average mortgage debt is $155,000.

WHAT IS LIFE? WHAT IS HAPPINESS?

Poverty moved to the suburbs with Meals-On-Wheels delivering food to those in need. "The Automatic Millionaire Homeowner" as they were called before 2008, ended up paying big money for the roof over their heads. Today they are "wrapped in debt like in silk robes."

LIVE BELOW YOUR MEANS AND NEEDS. OR, STRETCH YOUR FEET ACCORDING TO THE LENGTH OF YOUR CLOTH

"Stretch your feet according to the length of your cloth" is another wise Russian saying, or "Live below your means" which is an American saying.

Ted Turner liked to state on CNN how he respected money, starting from his teen years. As soon as he started working at age 21, for every $80 he made per week, he saved $10.

One judge on a popular *People's Court Show* advocated to her viewers to always live below their means, and she reinforced this point with her own personal example. When she began her career in New York City, she lived in a small rented studio apartment. She could not imagine wasting money on a bigger house (that to her had no value) instead of her own personal development (her career).

Also, please read my short story in this book, "What Is happiness? What Were the Happiest Years in Your life?" For me, it was when living in Africa. I was the only white woman living in an all-black neighborhood in Kinondoni in one small room that Mr. John Bosco gave to me and my child in his house, out of the goodness of his heart.

I had only 2 things in that room, a single bed that was falling apart and a child's crib. There was no telephone, no radio, and no TV. We were living on a $100 monthly stipend that my then husband received for his medical internship that he was completing at the Dar es Salam hospital. I did not know one word of English and taught it to myself from 6:00 a.m. to midnight.

But, I did not even notice my meager life. I was concentrating on only one objective—to learn English and get back to my engineering work and exciting life that was passing me by. Soon I learned English, went back to work, and regained my privileged life. While I was in Africa, those were the happiest years of my life.

☐ ☐ ☐

THE MORAL OF THE STORY

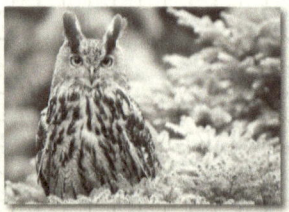

No money, no funny. The majority of people have no savings, but large debts. Nearly 36% of the people near retirement age have "0" money for retirement, according to the recent news reports. Today, the quality of life in the world and in the USA is in a downward spiral and is getting worse and worse every year. Unfortunately, this trend is not going to change. Ever. Why?

Just "look through the window" and see what is going on outside. The world has changed dramatically and become one single system—global capitalism—or "get rich quick from thin air."

What can one do? The downward trend is beyond your control. What is under your control is to stop spending and start saving money for a rainy day. Rent and do not buy, do not buy stuff that you can live without, stop wrapping yourself in debt as in silk robes and live below your means, or at least live according to your needs and not your wants.

If you are willing to do all of the above, you will become happy and prosperous. Grow up and become responsible for your life. Remember: "No money, no funny."

SHORT STORY #16

WHO ARE YOU?

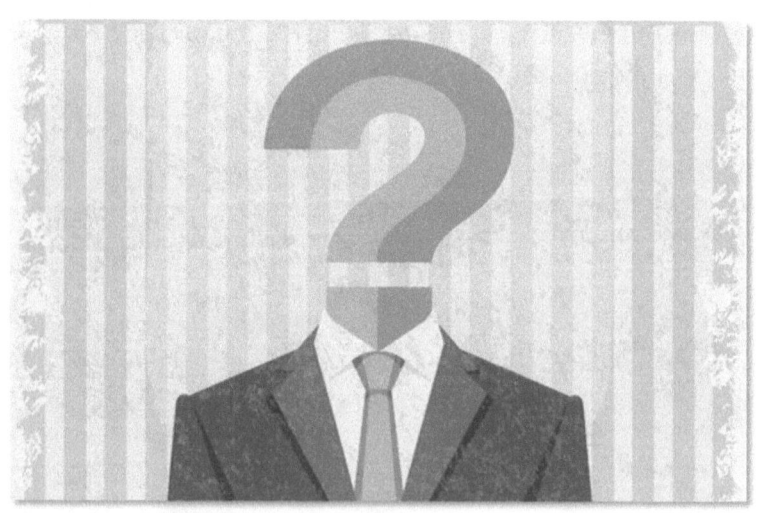

WHAT IS LIFE? WHAT IS HAPPINESS?

□ □ □

When I was a graduate student at Johns Hopkins University, I felt very comfortable doing math and science, which is why all my courses were quantitative. One semester, there was one very popular course among the students called "Personal Development."

Though popular, to me such a course was not a serious one. Many of the other students encouraged me to take the course, so, to be open minded, and out of curiosity, I went to the first lecture to see what it was all about—although I had already decided ahead of time that it was not for me and I was not going to take it. How wrong I was.

The professor started the lecture by writing a question across the blackboard: "Who are you?" Then, he went through the roll call asking each student to give a short answer to his question. He summarized them and wrote all their answers below the question. They were:

#1. I am a student.
#2. I am a son, a daughter—I have parents and siblings.
#3. I am a husband, a wife—I am married.
#4. I am a father, a mother—I have children.
#5. I am a professional—I work for company ABC.
#6. I am a homeowner—I have a house.

The professor read out the answers one by one, analyzed them, and then based on his knowledge and experience, concluded that all the students' answers were wrong. He crossed out each of the 6 summary answers. Across each wrong answer he gave his response—the correct, right answers based on facts and life's reality.

For the students' answer #1: "I am a student," he stated, "Yes, today, tomorrow, or the next year indeed you are a student. But your student status is a temporary one. In just 1–2 years, you are going to graduate and your student status will cease. So, who are you?" He again addressed his question to the students. There were no volunteers to challenge or contradict him.

For the students' answer #2: "I am a son, a daughter—I have parents and siblings," the professor declared, "Only one thing in life is constant—change. Today your parents and siblings are nice and great; they are supporting you. But tomorrow, or in a few years, everyone is going to change: your parents, your siblings—and you. There will be no more harmony, but a great discord in the family. All of you will be living in different parts of the country and will see each other seldom. Nothing lasts forever and eventually your parents will die. So, who are you?"

For the students' answer #3: "I am a husband, a wife—I am married," he had a statistical answer. "Statistics show that in the USA, the divorce rate is over 50%. So most people are eventually divorced. You cannot be sure that such a statistical probability will miss you."

WHAT IS LIFE? WHAT IS HAPPINESS?

For the students' answer #4: "I am a mother, a father—I have children," the professor said, "Your children will grow up. They are nice and cute when they are small. Once they are teens, they rebel against their parents. They may get out of control and bring you nothing but trouble. Once they become adults, you will be lucky if they remember you or call you sometimes. Even more, they will dump all their life problems on you and blame one person—you—because you are an easy scapegoat".

For the students' answer #5: "I am a professional—I work for company ABC," his answer was, "Your employment is temporary. You are employed as long as a company needs you and you are not creating problems for them and are making them a profit. Every company has many employees, just like you. You could get fired or laid off, the company could be bought by another company, it could shrink, or go bankrupt, and many more reasons."

For the students' answer #6: "I am a homeowner—I have a house" the professor also had a correct answer. "Your house is just a roof over your head and keeping it depends on luck. A tornado, hurricane, earthquake, mudslide, storm, fire, flood, wind, etc. could quickly reduce your house to a pile of rubbish. What if you get divorced, or get relocated? You would have to sell your house. Or what if you lose your job, or get sick and could no longer afford to pay your mortgage and other house expenses? The bank will repossess your house."

Next, he underlined the above questions and answers and wrote the same question again on another board: "Who are you?"

Confused, but in agreement with his realistic and cynical response to every question, we students had no other answers.

He gave us his answer: "Regardless of outside circumstances such as loss of job or a house, divorce, growing children, changed people, dead parents, or disagreement with siblings, only one thing remains constant and that is *you, yourself.*

"Look in a mirror. Your only wealth and assets are what you carry inside of you. Your knowledge, information, skills, and experiences are your wealth that you store in your brain's memory, and can take with you anywhere in the world. Your memory of information will help you to adopt, re-engineer, survive, and solve all of your life problems.

"There is only one person who can always help you in this world—you. Other people are temporary in your life and will, on occasion, give you temporary help. Other people and circumstances will change, regardless of your wishes and hopes to keep them on your side.

"There will only be one person in your life who is constantly with you solving your everyday problems, and that is you, yourself."

THE MORAL OF THE STORY

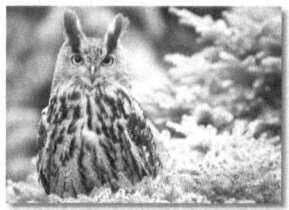

Question: Who are you? Answer: Physical possessions and people all are temporary in your life; they are outside of you. Invest in yourself, not in material possessions, because wealth is inside of you, not outside. It is located in the memories of your mind.[1]

You are what is stored in your brain's memory: your information, knowledge, skills, experiences, people you met and learned from, places you visited, books you read, courses you took, schools you went to, mentors you met, and friends you learned from.

The more knowledge and experiences you acquire, the more intelligent and sophisticated you become, and the greater probability you have to survive and succeed under difficult circumstances. By retrieving from your brain's database, you will find solutions to all of your personal and professional problems.

In short: The greatest wealth and assets you have reside inside of you. It is the database of knowledge that you have accumulated inside your brain that will help you deal with life's greatest challenges. Look forward, not back into the past, as one popular saying said: "Yesterday is history, tomorrow is a mystery, today is a gift, that is why it's called the present."

---

[1] Please read my other story in this book: "Our Mind Is a Tape Recorder."

SHORT STORY

#17

WHO IS MORE INTELLIGENT? A PERSON OR A COMPUTER?

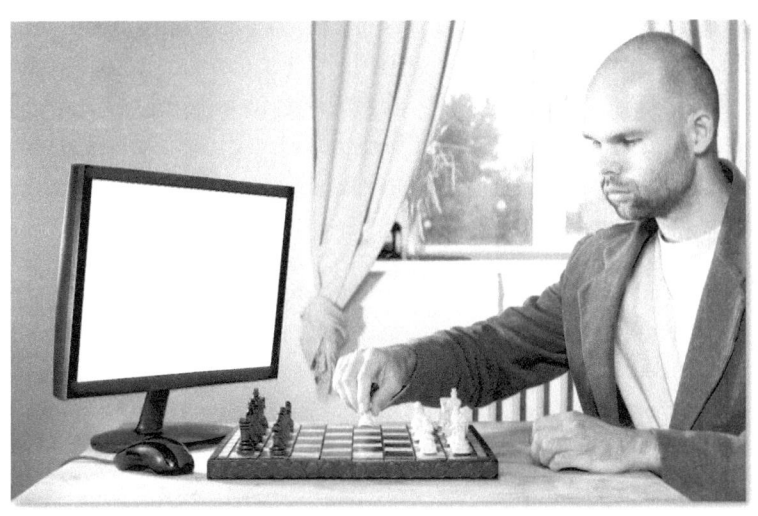

□ □ □

When teaching an undergraduate course at the university called "Information Systems," or "Computers," I noticed that my 21–22-year-old students were treating computers as if they were human beings, especially in the lab. Puzzled and curious to solve this mystery, I gave them a small test.

At the top of a blackboard, I wrote question #1 asking them: "Who is more intelligent—a computer or a person?" Below this question, using 2 axes (X and Y), I drew a scale from 0 to 10. I asked them where they would put computer intelligence on this scale. They raised their hands and gave the computer the highest intelligence marks, which were between 9 and 10. As for a person's intelligence? They were split between 2 and 4.

Laughing and giggling, I wrote the same question on the 2nd blackboard, except I substituted a computer for a car. Question #2 became, "Who is more intelligent—a car or a person?" They were confused. Why did I use such an analogy? To them it was obvious that a person is more intelligent than a car.

Then I explained that both a car and a computer have no intelligence; they are just machines. Both are innovations designed to solve people's needs for speed and convenience. Both were designed by engineers. Engineers designed cars for faster transportation; that is, to transport people from point A to point B faster than walking on foot or using a horse and carriage. Also designed for transportation are bikes, boats, ships, trains, and airplanes. Indeed, there is an analogy between a car and a computer because both have 2 components: hardware and software.

A car's hardware is its metal body, engine and parts, and like computer hardware, it is physical in nature. A car's software is its driver.

A driver is a logical person who makes a car run and he performs operations on the spot according to his needs: start, drive, slow, stop, reverse. The driver of a car performs *dynamic tasks*; he changes or modifies his personal driving needs on the spot, such as changing the gears from drive to park; from going forward to reverse, and others tasks.

A computer is also a machine, or a device, designed by engineers to satisfy people's needs, for fast electronic speed in doing everyday tasks such as: logging on to websites, filling out forms, calculating, typing, operating programs, generating reports, doing monthly billing and many more functions.

The computer, like a car, also has 2 main components: hardware and software. The hardware is physical in nature: there is a monitor, keyboard, mouse, hard drive, printer. The software or computer programs are logical in nature and are stored in the computer's memory.

These programs are usually written in high-level programming languages, and then interpreted into computer code. But, computer programs *are static*; they are already stored in the computer's memory and cannot be changed or modified on the spot by the person using the computer.

In summary, the analogy between a car and a computer is:

(1) Physical body: a car and a computer have physical parts (a car has a physical body, a computer has hardware).
(2) Logical commands to operate: a car has a driver, a computer has software.

A car cannot drive without a driver. A computer can not perform tasks without software. The car driver performs *dynamic (changing) tasks* to drive a car: start, drive, stop, and he changes the tasks constantly according to his or her needs.

A computer operator (a person) can't perform any tasks without having software instructions (a driver) installed on his computer. Except, software, or programs, *are static;* they are already stored in the computer's memory and cannot be changed or modified on the spot by a person using a computer.

To simplify: driving a car is dynamic and driving tasks are changed on the spot; computer software is static and cannot be changed on the spot.

WHAT IS LIFE? WHAT IS HAPPINESS?

All the time, people have been curious about a computer replacing the human mind and they have tried to design and replicate it. They have come to the conclusion that it is impossible, even if they designed an enormous computer.

There is nothing that can replace a human mind's enormous intellectual and logical capacity. The human mind is dynamic, flexible, and can solve various problems immediately, simultaneously, and on the spot. Not the computer; even if they designed an enormous one with thousands of software programs inside, it could never replicate the human mind.

It was my young, undergraduate students who thought that a computer was more intelligent than people. What about adults, what do they think? Recently I found the answer.

On a major TV network, a discussion between middle-aged adults, a newsman and "an expert" was held. The expert held on to his belief, postulating that some computers are more intelligent than people. To prove his discoveries, he referred to some computer and software names. That was bizarre.

Before the personal computer was invented, many other devices were used for calculations—the abacus to add and subtract figures, then mechanical machines to crunch the numbers. The logarithmic scale, or the slide ruler, was an essential tool for engineers to perform functions such as logarithms, roots, and trigonometry, but was not used for addition and subtraction.

After World War II, computers of immense sizes were invented for the defense industry and for engineering companies; at that time, computers were big in size, about the size of a huge room. The 1970s saw a renaissance of many personal computer versions, but it was not until the user-friendly computer, called the Apple II, that sales picked up and later sold on a mass scale.

There is a computer rule, "Garbage in, garbage out," which is widely used in information systems and in engineering companies. What does this rule mean? This rule could also be applicable to personal computing, especially any time a person is filling some input variables into a table to receive the probability result.

To demonstrate this rule, let's consider a visual example of one specific program that calculates how many calories per day a person should consume to maintain good health.

To solve the problem, to find the number of calories a person should consume per day, an appropriate program is used. The program has a table asking one to input some variables such as age, gender, weight, height, then press the button "calculate" and on the next page get a result, the number of calories this particular person needs to consume. Variables in this problem are simple and familiar and very few errors should occur.

Now, just for demonstration, let's make an error in just one input variable, say the person's age; the output the computer would give would be wrong for this particular person. This "Garbage in, garbage out" rule applies here. The probability of getting the wrong output, or "garbage out," increases tremendously with the complexity of the problem.

Now let's take another, more difficult problem from engineering to calculate the amount of stress a steel beam experiences from holding a ceiling up in an apartment building.

The input variables an engineer needs to know are the dead loads from the reinforced concrete ceiling, from the structures above, and from the beam itself and live loads from the tenant's furniture, appliances, and people.

All those inputs are just approximate numbers based on this particular engineer's previous experiences and his logic and common sense. Imagine if an engineer made an error with just one variable, the output would be wrong and potentially catastrophic; the beam would crack and fail and then a part or the whole building would collapse.

Engineers almost never make errors. Why? 1st they calculate by hand the approximate output, a beam's stresses in this example, then they compare it to a computer's output. If both results do not match, they find the error and recalculate the beam's stresses again.

THE MORAL OF THE STORY

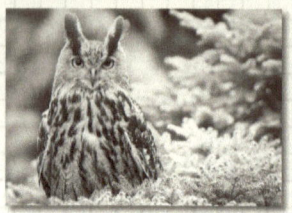

Who is more intelligent? A person or a computer? The innovation of computers has contributed to the quality of life of today's civilization. Computers speed up calculations, research, and getting everyday tasks done and obtain information for almost every subject or idea.

Today, computers are an everyday tool. But a computer is just that—a tool—that was designed to ease people's lives in performing everyday tasks and solve problems.

People have always been curious to develop a computer that could replace or replicate the human mind, but as of today, it has not yet materialized.

A person's mind can perform amazements and the depth of knowledge, skills, and information stored in a human brain is just someone's guess. The brain is dynamic, logical, and flexible, and it can solve problems on the spot and simultaneously. A computer cannot do this.

Here is a tip. When using software programs for calculations, always keep in mind one important computer law—"garbage in, garbage out." Just one wrong variable or input will produce the wrong output.

SHORT STORY

#18

MY 2-YEAR-OLD GRANDSON PARIS' WORLD

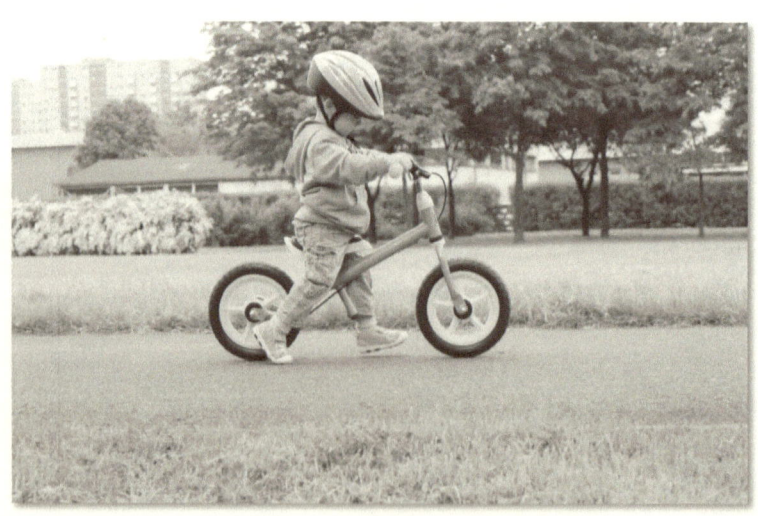

WHAT IS LIFE? WHAT IS HAPPINESS?

□ □ □

The morning was still very dark when I woke up. I stretched like a cat and felt very happy. I had no responsibility. I was on vacation and had come back to spend some time with my 2-year-old grandson Paris.

Curiously, I looked forward to uncovering the mysteries of the breaking day. The clock indicated it was past 6:00 a.m. in San Francisco. "Oh, I overslept," I thought.

Then I decided to read some magazines in the living room. Such a journey presented some small challenges. Afraid to wake anyone, I tiptoed to the living room, navigating 2 squeaky doors and a very long corridor. Acknowledging my presence, the hardwood floor noisily answered *Rep... Rep...Rep* to the pressure of my steps.

As I reached the end of the corridor, I made a pleasant discovery. In the living room, an earlier bird was already playing his video game, my 2-year-old grandson Paris.

Amused, I leaned against the wall and looked at him. He planted his little body in the middle of the huge, green sofa that perfectly matched his eyes. His golden curls, like a bunch of sunflowers, stretched in all directions. His long, thin neck tilted towards the TV. A light-colored t-shirt exposed his arms, which had several peeling temporary tattoos I had given him yesterday. A large pillow completely covered his legs, his 2 bare feet sticking out. Both hands held a remote control on top of the pillow.

He completely ignored my presence. I am sure he heard me before I saw him because of the noises I made as I walked to the living room from my bedroom. I peeled myself from the wall and, as I crossed his view, greeted him: "Good morning, Paris." To my greeting, he firmly replied, "Go away!"

Caught off guard by such a naughty response, I sat on another sofa and thought about this little rascal. During my scrutiny, he did not change his pose, but continued looking straight at the TV screen, watching me through the corner of his eye.

He woke up moody, was the first thought that crossed my mind. And his little mind probably designed some powerful antics for me, his grandma. Now he had a chance to test his power over me. And with his "Go away!" he was testing how far he could push his grandma and get away with it.

But then I started guessing and wondering further. Whose personality had he inherited? Where had he learned those words? Why had he said it?

My mind searched for reasons. Paris carries a kaleidoscope of his ancestors' genes, I thought. His grandparents came from different continents and have different nationalities. Their physical characteristics, personalities, temperaments, creativities, gifts, interests, and habits were mixed into an amalgam and produced him, one unique and special person.

WHAT IS LIFE? WHAT IS HAPPINESS?

Adding to this is the external environment in which he grew. Every day, thousands of pieces of information bombarded his tender mind.

I was wondering why children with the same parents were so different and opposite. At this young age, no one knew whose genes Paris would inherit. After I did this inheritance inventory, I felt a bit better.

And I thought about more reasons...Nothing happens by accident. There is a reason for that, I thought. My little grandson said, "Go away!" to me not by accident; it had a purpose. He probably tried to communicate that he has a desire, the same as every adult, to be alone.

When a child is alone, he can mature, develop, and grow his mind. That is why impulses propelled him to wake up early this morning to watch his video while the adults were asleep. That way he had an opportunity to learn wonderful things about the fascinating world around without an adult's interference and interruption.

And though I am a loving and generous grandma, I am still a dominant adult who does not want to leave him alone. I interrupted his world, his learning process. I should learn to respect his child's world and give him an opportunity to mature in it. At the age of 2, Paris has already developed his identity. He has a set of feelings and sees the world in his personal and unique way.

Besides all the above reasoning, my ego dictated that I should let him know that his naughty behavior was not appreciated. Soon I had such an opportunity.

Paris jumped from the sofa and, in the quick succession of a pro, performed several operations at once. He ejected a video, inserted a new one, turned off the TV, then turned it on and adjusted the sound and focus. I was stunned to see how his 2-year-old mind could master and perform all the operations at once and correctly.

Soon, Paris had enough of his video. His curiosity turned to another person in the room—me. He was no longer ignoring me and instead signaled that he wanted to communicate. I welcomed the opportunity and suggested reading him a book.

Without a word, still projecting his maturity and independence, he left the sofa in the living room and disappeared into his playroom. Soon he appeared with *The Big Red Dog* and sat next to me to signal that I could start reading from page #1. I obliged.

He knew the story well. He took control of my reading, flipping pages to indicate silently where I should read. I had no problem until the last page. Here was an opportunity to teach him that naughty behavior, such as telling grandma to "Go away!" is not rewarded.

On the last page, a big dog named Clifford was stretched across 2 pages. Clifford held a man's shoe in his mouth. At the bottom of the page was a skinny, distracted man, a shoe cobbler. He ran out of his shop, very angry that Clifford had stolen his shoe.

Seizing the opportunity, I did not follow the script on this last page, but instead invented and improvised my own. I emphasized that Clifford was a bad dog because he had stolen the shoe from the cobbler. Such bad behavior should never be rewarded.

With gusto, my voice raised, my finger pointed and shaking in the air, I said: "No! No! No! Clifford! You are a very bad and a naughty dog. You did a very bad thing. You stole my shoe!" I looked at Paris to see if my message got across. He was smiling with sparkles in his eyes. Clearly he understood my message.

Later that evening, Paris came to me like a cat. He rubbed his little body against my feet, pressed his arms against my lap and with twinkles in his eyes, softly asked, "Grandma, read me a book." "All right," I said. Humming something, he galloped into his playroom that was overstuffed with toys, fuzzy animals, games, and books. Somehow he found the same book, *The Big Red Dog*.

Only this time he did not want me to read from the beginning. Instead, he went directly to the script of interest—he opened it on the last page. And, as before, I took on Clifford the Dog.

This time I gave an even better performance. Shaking my finger I yelled, "No! No! No! Clifford! You are a very bad and a naughty dog; you did a very bad thing. You stole my shoe!" Paris' eyes flicked and a broad smile brought dimples to his cheeks. He understood perfectly what I was up to. There was harmony between us. Without exchanging words, we understood each other.

Many studies were conducted on grandparents' genes skipping a generation and resurfacing in their grandchildren's genes. Even plants, as one recent experiment reports, took normal genes carried by their grandparents by bypassing genetic abnormalities carried by both parents. That is why grandparents and grandchildren can get along very well and understand each other. They have a lot in common; namely, they have the same genes.

A week later, flying back to my new home in Tampa, Florida, I noticed a few small children around Paris' age. On my numerous other flights, I am sure, there had been small children. But I did not remember ever noticing them.

This flight was different. The sea of noises and words, like the sounds of a jungle at night, came from 200 people on the plane. No single sound attracted my attention except one. Predominant and familiar to me, the phrase, "Go away!" popped out.

I located the source. Not far behind me, a small boy about Paris' age and height was sandwiched between his parents. In front of him, on the arm table, some colorful game pieces were laid out. Competing with each other, his doting parents were trying to help him advance in his game. The little boy kept yelling, "Go away!" our entire journey. I smiled and giggled.

□ □ □

THE MORAL OF THE STORY

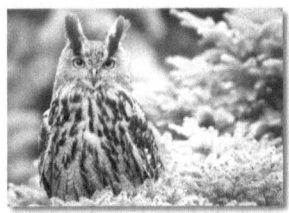

When I became a grandmother, suddenly from everywhere small children began entering my domain. Their existence is amplified and attracts my attention. My 2-year-old grandson Paris' world is popping up into mine.

SHORT STORY

#19

WHAT IS A LIFE SPAN?
WHY MAN-MADE THINGS DEPRECIATE AND NOT APPRECIATE?

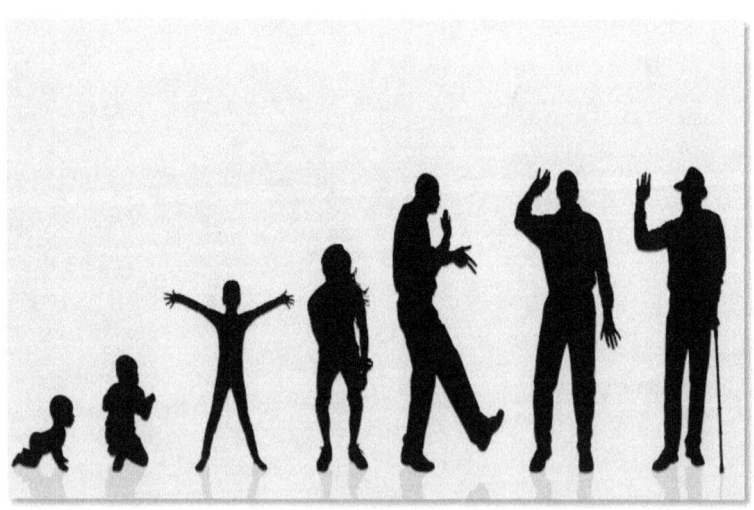

WHAT IS LIFE? WHAT IS HAPPINESS?

□ □ □

What is a life span? A life span is the length of time a person or animal lives or man-made things function. Nature is eternal or lives forever. Humans have a life expectancy. All man-made things around us have a life span.

Nature has eternity, or endless life. The Earth is 4.5 billion years old and it will continue living forever because it is eternal. The Amazon River is 11 million years old. The Pacific Ocean is 180 million years old. The Rolling Hills in Rwanda, Africa, are 700 million years old. The longest river in the world, the Nile in Africa, is many millions of years old. It originates in Rwanda, flows up to Northern Egypt, and empties into the Mediterranean Sea. Lake Baikal is the oldest, largest, and deepest freshwater lake in the world; it is 25 million years old and is located in Siberia, Russia.

Humans also have a life expectancy. Humans do not live forever, nor do they get younger with age. Instead, they get older. Their bodies wear down, all their organs deteriorate and the body eventually dies.

What is a life expectancy? It is a statistically projected number of years which indicates a person's length of life.

An average life expectancy is the time between birth and death. In the 18th century, the average human life expectancy was 35 years; in the 19th century, it was 48 years of age. Today, the life expectancy in Monaco is 87, in

Sweden it is 83, in Canada it is 82, in the USA it is 79, in Russia it is 70. In less developed nations, life expectancy is low. For example, in Africa today, the average life expectancy is 45 years.

All man-made things around us have a life span. Engineers design man-made things. Some examples are cars, computers, TVs, kitchen appliances, bridges, buildings, single houses, and many other things around us.

Those things are all designed to last a certain numbers of years, called life spans. What is the life span for man-made things? It is the length of time for which man-made things were designed to function.

The length of the life span of things depends on the strength of the materials that were used to build or manufacture things. For example, cars were designed to last for 10 years on average, desktop computers for 3–5 years, dishwashers and microwave ovens designed for 5 years, and refrigerators and electric ranges for 10 years. Reinforced concrete bridges are designed for 45 years on average. Reinforced concrete apartment buildings are designed for 25 years, and commercial reinforced concrete buildings for 37 years.

Single-family dwellings made from plywood frames are designed for a "0" year life span because they will stay erect only until the 1st tornadoes, mudslides, floods, fires, hurricanes, strong winds, bring them down.

WHAT IS LIFE? WHAT IS HAPPINESS?

Could engineers design things with much longer life spans? Yes, they could, but the cost would rise astronomically. With age, all things deteriorate and decay from weather, wear out from wear and tear, and stop functioning or fall apart. That is why all things depreciate with age rather than appreciate.

For example, a new car, such as a Toyota, costs $20,000 brand new in a show room. However, as soon as a buyer purchases that Toyota and drives it off the lot, it starts depreciating. At the age of 3, the Toyota costs $10,000, at 10 years $3,000 and at 15 years $200 or basically nothing.

To find a price for any type of car, new or old, there are some popular car websites; one of them is the "Kelly Blue Book" website. This typical example applies to all man-made things. All things around us—cars, computers, kitchen appliances, bridges, buildings, single-family dwellings, and many more—depreciate, not appreciate.

Common sense dictates that the same depreciation rule should apply to the housing industry. No, not for the real estate industry. Real estate changed the "depreciation" law into the "appreciation" law for buildings and single-family homes to fit their "get rich quick" objectives. According to the real estate industry, as commercial buildings, apartments/condos, and single-family houses age, they "appreciate." When cars depreciate; no one disagrees with that law.

Why is there such an opposite discrepancy? That did not happen by accident. There is a reason for that. You see, the real estate industry is the most secretive industry and they do not have, as cars do, a Kelly Blue Book website to find the real structural value of apartments, condos, and houses according to their age. They spend millions of dollars every year marketing and programming the population into thinking that apartments/condos and single-family houses "appreciate" and that owning a house is "the American dream."

The state governments knew that, for example, condos depreciated with age and that they should be priced accordingly based on their age. In order to protect condo buyers, the states therefore issued laws and regulations governing the sale of condos in their states.

The laws require that a condo seller must send to a condo buyer a statement certificate via registered mail stating how many years of structural life are left in that particular condo. How does one calculate a structural life? It is very simple, as shown below:

A) Given facts:
1. A reinforced concrete condo/apartment building is designed to last for 25 years, it is a public information.
2. From city buildings records it is easy to find out in what year any particular building of condos/apartments was built, for example, in 1995.

3. It is obvious in what year this particular condo was put up for sale, for example, in 2014.

B) How many years of structural life are left in this particular condo as of 2014?

C) Calculate:
   1) How old is this condo?
      (2014 put up for sale–1995 year was built)=19 years old.
   2) How many years of structural life are left in this condo?
      (25 years life span–19 years old)=6 years.

The calculations above show that this condo has only 6 years of structural life left in it. Let's apply this analogy to a car, a new Chevrolet, which costs $13,000 brand new. Assume a Chevrolet was built to have a 7–8 year life span. Today, it is 17 years old with little to no structural life left in it. Knowing this information, a buyer can go to various car websites and find the price for a 17-year-old Chevrolet, which is $100 or nothing. The point is: an old Chevrolet depreciates and does not appreciate! No one will pay the same price for a 17-year-old Chevrolet as he would for a new Chevrolet.

How many condo buyers knew about the above state's law? Very few, or none. I personally have never met even one condo buyer who knows about this state law. If condo buyers knew about it, their common sense would dictate that they seek a decent price.

For a 15-year-old condo, the price should only be ⅓ or less than the price of a new condo; and for a 25-year-old condo, a few thousand dollars (it has zero years of structural life), provided that condos/apartments were designed and built as reinforced concrete buildings with a 25-year-life span and were not built from plywood frame that has no structural life.

One does not need to be a rocket scientist to figure out that similarity or analogy exists between a car and a condo. Why then is the reality just the opposite? In 2014, a condo buyer will pay a much higher price for a 19-year-old condo than the price was for this particular condo when it was new. In 1995, when the condos were built and housing was in a dead zone, this new condo was sold for $25,000. In 2014, or 19 years later, this old condo now is selling for $200,000, or 800% more. Why?

Single-family dwellings/house. As for the single-family dwellings, the reality is even worse than it is for condos. Let's repeat it again—a single-family home has a structural life of "0" years. This is all because its structure was not built from reinforced concrete materials to withstand tornadoes, mudslides, rain, winds, hurricanes, fires, floods, and the rapid decay of plywood. It was built out of plywood, so a single-family dwelling was designed to survive on sheer luck and some prayers.

You still do not believe that a single-family dwelling, like a car, does depreciate, not appreciate? Then let's look at what the "appreciation value" of this house is after tornadoes, mudslides, hurricanes, winds, floods, fires. What is left from a single-family house is a pile of rubbish because pieces of the wood/house blew away with the wind.

Moreover, those wooden strips that are left in a rubbish pile are old, crushed, and decayed pieces of wood; they are not gold strips that would sell at an appreciated value. The aftermath of Hurricane Sandy in 2012 is one such classic example.

But this would not happen to apartments/condos if they were built from reinforced concrete materials. Natural disasters can damage their windows and some doors, but would not be able to smash the reinforced concrete buildings into a pile of rubbish (as it did single-family homes) because the building's main structure would be able to stand up to the natural disaster. As the example indicates after Hurricane Sandy in 2012, apartments buildings were standing up and renters were continue living in them.

One more important point or fact to question and know when buying a condo or renting an apartment is this—was the 2–5 story apartment/condo, or high-rise building built from reinforced concrete materials, or just from plywood, as in single-family houses?

An example to emphasize this point occurred in March 2014 when for a few days, local and national TV stations broadcast a spectacular fire at a condo building in the San Francisco Mission district.

A massive fire destroyed the $227 million high-rise construction project of 360 apartments/condos. Not even 150 firefighters could save it; they kept out of the inferno. The truth was, only the lower 2 floors were made of reinforced concrete; the rest of the upper floors were plywood. Fire quickly incinerated the plywood, and debris collapsed the structure. The fire's intensity threatened buildings across the street, where windows broke from the heat.

In this $227 million building, the price for each condo was $630,000. It was a building developer's scam, and his objective was to get rich quick by building a high-rise building from wood, not from reinforced concrete. Why?

The wood structure would cost a fraction of the cost for reinforced concrete. To build a 1-bedroom condo from wood would have cost probably $20,000–$30,000. This developer already was selling those plywood condos for $630,000 each, before he even finished his construction. His profit was 20–30 times more than it cost to build! This is simply a case of deceit and avarice!

Even more, let's imagine if these fires had started after this high-rise plywood building was occupied with condo owners. How many of them would have escaped the inferno? Not many, and the majority of the occupants would have died inside.

□ □ □

THE MORAL OF THE STORY

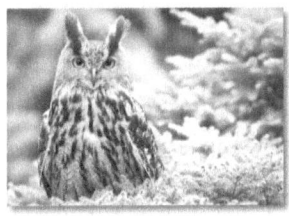

What is a life span? Everything has a life span. Even humans do not live forever, nor do they get younger with age. Instead, they get old with age. Their bodies wear down, all the organs deteriorate and the body eventually dies. On average, the life expectancy of a person is 45 years (in Africa) and is 70–85 years (in Europe and the USA).

The exact same law can be applied to man-made things, such as: cars, computers, TVs, dishwashers, refrigerators, microwave oven, bridges, reinforced concrete apartments and commercial buildings, and single-family dwellings because man-made things also depreciate with age! Common sense dictates that the same law should also apply to single-family housing. A house, like a car, depreciates and does not appreciate!

The difference is: to find the real price or depreciation price for a car, one can go to car websites, such as the Kelly Blue Book website, and voila, find the depreciated price of a car. Why do such websites not exist for housing? The answer is very simple: a lot of money and marketing is spent to keep homeowners from finding out this information. The real estate industry is highly secretive; they spend millions of dollars every year to market, program, and indoctrinate people into believing that an older house appreciates, and a single-family dwelling made from plywood is "the American dream."

SHORT STORY #20

ONLY ONE THING IN LIFE IS CONSTANT—CHANGE. OR, RISE, FALL, AND DISAPPEARANCE OF EMPIRES AND POWERFUL COUNTRIES

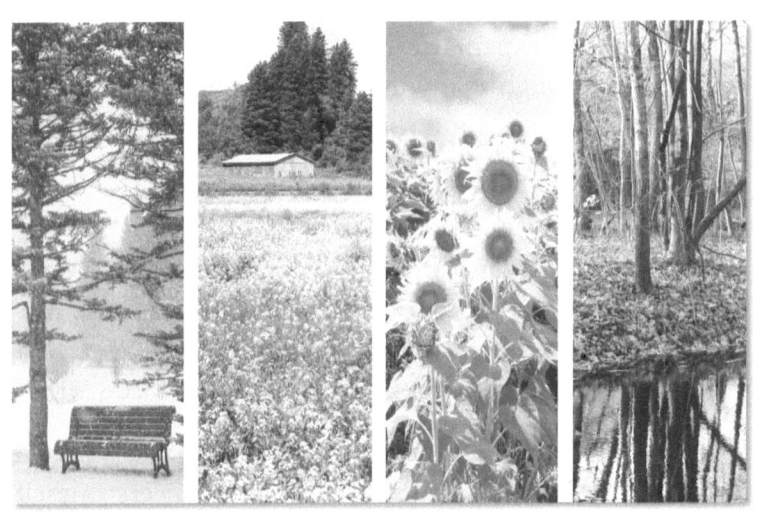

□ □ □

"What is constant in life?" was a question that Dr. Raven, one of the professors and the mentor in my doctoral program, asked his students. "Nothing, except—change. Only one thing in life is constant—change," he answered. Students did not disagree with him.

Personal changes, changes in the world, changes inside the country all are constantly bombarding and alarmed people and are transforming their attitudes, beliefs, and lives. What are those changes? How do we live and survive in such an unpredictable changing world? At the end of this story, will be the answer.

I) CHANGES IN PEOPLE: PEOPLE LIVED, WORKED, AND THEN DIED

Average people experience hundreds of changes in their lifetime, go through many events and circumstances—the majority of them beyond their control—constantly living under enormous stress, anxiety and many suffer life-threatening events.

How does a person survive in a such stressful and threatening time? By progression. He progresses constantly and develops his intellect from a child to a teenager, to a young adult, to a middle-aged adult, and to a wise senior.

He acquires new information, knowledge, new skills, and constantly adapts, adjusts, and re-engineers oneself according to internal and external changes and events that are taking place in the outside world and inside environment.

The more knowledge, information, and skills a person has stored in his brain's memory, the greater chance he has for survival. That is: the more intellectual a person becomes, the easier it is for him to live and survive.

Even more, a person's life has 2 limitations: (1) His short life span; and (2) His physical and mental body deterioration due to age. He spends a considerable amount of energy and time counter-balancing those 2 limitations.

(1) The short life span (life expectancy). Everything has a life span. Computers are designed for 3 years, appliances for 5 years, cars for 10 years, reinforced concrete apartments buildings for 25 years, bridges for 43 years. Dogs live 10 years and cats 15 years. Some trees live thousands of years. The Pacific Ocean plate is as old as the Earth is. The Earth is 4.5 billion years old; it will continue living forever, and has eternal life. The average life expectancy today for Africans is 45 years; for Americans 79 years; for Europeans 84 years; for Russians 70 years.

(2) The physical and mental body deteriorates due to age. A person's rapid physical and mental growth progresses up to age 25–27, on average, after which time it begins slowing down and deteriorating.

By age 40, many functions have already slowed down and by age 60, a person has lost 50% of muscle strength, hearing and vision, and certain congenital illnesses may begin to take root.

At the same time, the outside world is changing constantly and pressing a person to change, adopt, and re-engineer himself in order to survive.

II) CHANGES IN CIVILIZATIONS: CIVILIZATIONS LIVED, PROSPERED, AND MYSTERIOUSLY DISAPPEARED

Many ancient civilizations mysteriously disappeared: the Mayan civilization (from Mexico to Guatemala); Indus Valley (India, Pakistan, Iran, Afghanistan); Polynesian (Islands in Pacific Ocean); Cahokia (North America); Khmer Empire (Cambodia); Aksum Empire (Ethiopia); Inca Civilization (Peru), and many more.

III) CHANGES IN MODERN POWERFUL COUNTRIES: THEIR RISE, FALL, AND DISAPPEARANCE

During the modern period, nations and empires rose to power, dominated the world for many years, or centuries, then fell and disappeared. Some examples:[1]

FRANCE, 1450S–1815

Was a dominant empire that conquered many colonies around the world. In 1800–1814, French Emperor Napoleon Bonaparte had a military ambition to spread France's dominance further to conquer the whole European and Russian Empire. After Napoleon's disastrous invasion of Russia in 1812, he abdicated and was sent into exile on the island of Elba.

The French Revolution of 1789 transformed France's monarchy into a New Republic; it had many mottos, and one main motto: Liberté, Égalité, Fraternité [Liberty, Equality, Fraternity (brotherhood)] for all people.

Later, revolutionaries stormed the Bastille and executed the King and sent Marie Antoinette to the guillotine. Accomplishments of French Revolution: French monarchy was abolished; Napoleon Bonaparte rose to power; declaration of rights of man and the citizens.

SAFAVID EMPIRE, 1501–1736
Was a very important ruling empire of Iran. They spread Shi'a Islam in Iran, Caucasus area, and in Central and South Asia to the present era.

DUTCH REPUBLIC, 1581–1795
After achieving independence from Spain, the Dutch Republic blossomed into the Dutch Golden Age; their skills in shipping and trading, science and art were the most acclaimed in the world.

EARLY BRITISH EMPIRE, 1600–1815
Through growth in trade with India and the Far East, British began colonizing overseas colonies. At its peak it was the most powerful and the largest empire in the world

with colonies in Canada, India, the Caribbean, Australia and New Zealand, and some colonies in Africa. It was once said that the sun never set on the British Empire.

MUGHAL EMPIRE, 1526–1857
Was imperial power from Uzbekistan, Timurid descendant of Timur and Genghis Khan, established the Mughal Empire that ruled 1/4 of the world population and lasted 300 years.

EARLY OTTOMAN EMPIRE, 1400S–1815
Was Islamic power and a Turkic state that constantly challenged Western Europe, and spanned across 3 continents of Southeast Europe, the Middle East and North Africa.

EARLY SPANISH EMPIRE, 1492–1815
Europe's foremost power in global trade routes and exploration, dominated the oceans and battlefields, and maintained one of the largest empires in the world.

MOSCOVITE RUSSIA, IMPERIAL RUSSIAN EMPIRE, THE SOVIET UNION EMPIRE, 1147–1991
Began in 14th century by Peter the Great period, 1672–1725, became the largest state in the world. 3 times the size of Europe, 2.5 time of the USA and the largest country in the world covering 1/6 of earth's mass, stretched from the Baltic Sea to the Pacific Ocean.

WHAT IS LIFE? WHAT IS HAPPINESS?

It has 11 different time zones; if one is in the West (in Murmansk) there is a sunrise and in the East (Vladivostok) is a sunset.

IV) CHANGES IN THE WORLD AFTER WORLD WAR II

The Soviet Union defeated Hitler in World War II, 1941–1945; saved Europe and humanity from Fascism. It expanded its dominance by adding Eastern Europe (Bulgaria, Romania, Czechoslovakia, Poland, Hungary, Albania, East Germany, and Yugoslavia) under its socialism umbrella. Socialism spread across the globe to China, India, Africa, Asia, Cuba, and South America.

The Soviet Union's influence grew and its socialist ideas, like wild fire, spread across the globe. Some of the benefits of socialism were: equal opportunity for all; women were equal to men in voting, in education, in work; 4-month maternity leave and free childcare for women; free health care, education and cheap housing for all citizens; labor laws (8 hour workday); prohibition of child labor; safe working conditions; sick leaves; 2–4 weeks of vacation time; pensions and benefits.

After World War II, Western Europe and Britain were weak militarily, economically, and morally. In this environment, it was not by accident that colonial uprisings began against West European powers. In 1947, India gained its independence from Britain; the Chinese Revolution of 1949 overthrew the monarchy, and Mao Zedong's revolutionaries started building socialism; colonialism in Africa fell in the 1960s.

CHANGES: THE USA BECAME THE WORLD SUPERPOWER AFTER WORLD WAR II

The USA was the greatest beneficiary of World War II, 1941–1945. World War II transformed backward, agricultural, separatist USA that had no regular army and was in economic depression (the Great Depression of the 1930s) into a world superpower. How? Factories began working to produce arms and supplies for the war, American men enlisted to fight in the war, unemployment went down, and the Great Depression dwindled.

In June 1944, the Soviet Union, after 3 years of World War II on Russian soil, defeated Hitler, liberated itself and Europe, and the Soviet Red Army began marching on Berlin. At that point, afraid that now the Soviet Union would take Western Europe into its sphere of influence, the USA and the Britain in June 1944 opened the second front, called the Normandy Landing. The truth was, that during the first 3 years of World War II, the Soviet Union asked many times for the USA and Britain to stop the Russian bleeding and to open the second front. They refused, citing that they were too weak to fight Germans. On May 2, 1945, the Soviet Army conquered Berlin, and on May 9, 1941, there was a victory day. Germany capitulated; World War II was over.

The Soviet Union was leveled during 3 years of vicious fighting on Russian soil. After the war starvation and diseases descended upon the vulnerable Russian population. For the next 15–20 years, the Soviet Union was rebuilding the nation with mostly women and old men. Europe was also in ruins.

After the war, the Europeans began rebuilding from the war's devastation and were fighting starvation and diseases too. In 1948, the USA established the Marshal Plan to feed the starving Western Europeans.

Casualties in World War II: 26.6 million Russians were killed, almost all men between the age of 18 to 50; 405,399 Americans were killed, and 382,700 British. After the war Americans and British re-wrote history claiming they won World War II, not the Soviet Union.

After World War II, hundreds of thousands of engineers, scientists, and intellectuals left devastated Europe for the USA, as did all German specialists. They created many new industries. The USA, unscathed after the war, had no completions, grew enormously by producing goods for the world over. This propelled the USA to become the world superpower it is today.

CHANGES: THE BRITISH EMPIRE DISINTEGRATED AFTER WORLD WAR II

If before 1947 someone told the British that soon their Empire would be disintegrated, lose all its colonies, their standard of living would be plundered, the majority of the people would not be able to find jobs, their capitalist economy would dissolve and that Greater Britain would became "a sick man of Europe," they would never have believed it. Great Britain was "a sick man of Europe"—this label was given to Britain by the European Press for many years, from the 1950s–1990s.

How did Britain survive in the end? It changed its existing capitalist market economy into a new, mixed economy, a mixture of capitalism with socialism. It "did not reinvent the wheel," but due to its close proximity to Europe, it imported some of the European features of socialist economy, applicable to Britain's new changes—a mixed economic system.

CHANGES: FRANCE LOST ITS EMPIRE AFTER WORLD WAR II

In the 19th centuries, the French Empire was 1 of the 4 the largest in the world, behind the British Empire, the Russian Empire, and the Spanish Empire.

Soon after World War II, France lost all their vast colonies throughout the world. France had many colonies on all 6 continents—some were countries, and some were part of countries located in Europe, in South America, Africa, Asia, and Oceania.

V) CHANGES: OIL SHOCK. THE OIL EMBARGO OF 1973–1974 AND THE RISE OF OPEC

The Oil Embargo of 1973–74 sent a shock wave throughout the world. Especially hard hit were the USA, Western

Europe, and Africa. Their economies plunged, national wealth decreased sharply, and OPEC (Organization of Petroleum Exporting Countries) started "swimming in wealth." Before the Oil Embargo, gasoline prices in the USA were cheap, $0.25 per gallon; afterwards the price went sharply up.

Western Europe, which lost its colonies after World War II, had no gasoline or raw resources, and was buying all its necessities on the world market. It cut all economic aid to Africa.

Africa was devastated. Why did the Oil Embargo have such a dramatic impact on the African continent? In the 1960s, Africa got rid of colonialism and, one by one 50 or so countries became independent. The Oil Embargo quadrupled oil prices and Western Europe and the USA cut foreign aid to Africa. All specialists left Africa, construction stopped, factories ran out of parts and supplies, and hospitals had no medications. Soon jungles over grew the abandoned factories while crime skyrocketed. African progress stopped.

In China, India, Eastern Europe, and in some of South America the oil embargo had no effect. They were not buying oil from OPEC. Their currency was closed; they had a planned socialist economy: the people lived by needs not by wants, and lived below their means. They were trading only among themselves, and they had very few private cars to worry about gasoline prices.

VI) CHANGES: THE RUSSIAN AND THE SOVIET UNION 700-YEAR-OLD EMPIRE DISINTEGRATED IN 1991

The Soviet Union's 700-year-old empire disintegrated in 1991, which shifted the world into one single system—global capitalism—and pushed the USA and Western Europe down the hill.

Before the Soviet Union's disintegration, the world was simple—it was divided into 2 systems. Capitalism was represented by the USA, as the leader, with Western Europe, Canada and Japan as followers. Socialism was represented by the Soviet Union and China, India, Africa, Asia, Cuba, and South America—all were under the Soviet Union's umbrella.

Socialist countries all lived below their means, they did not trade with the Western World, and their currencies were "national and closed" (you could not exchange their currencies on a stock exchange—it had no value).

Before 1991, only the USA and Western Europe, Canada, and Japan (comprising 700 million people approximately) were buying oil and raw resources on the world market. Today over 7.2 billion people are buying, or 11 times more, fearlessly buying and competing with each other. The USA imports oil and many raw resources and paying for it over $2 trillion annually for those goods.

WHAT IS LIFE? WHAT IS HAPPINESS?

The American middle class, the heart of this nation, disappeared; today 1 in 2 Americans are in poverty or near poverty. Only the crooks on Wall Street, bankers, and the CEOs are multi-millionaires, and they keep inventing innovations on how to rob the population and the USA.

The world population is mushrooming. Everyone wants to be rich and "get rich quick from thin air." World habitants, over 7.2 billion of them, threatens to destroy our planet resulting in an ecological holocaust. They consumed almost all of the world's oil and raw resources, more cars are produced every minute, and more carbon monoxide is discharged into the air.

The North Pole is melting rapidly, and thousand of species have disappeared forever. The temperature is extremely hot and extremely cold, drought and floods, and extreme numbers of tornadoes, hurricanes, and fires destroying land, homes, and properties. Millions are starving from hunger, malnutrition, and diseases with no food, water, or shelters.

The best years are behind the USA and the West; they are bankrupt and sinking. They cannot compete with the global capitalism that is growing.

Today China took over the USA and became the #1 economy in the world. Now, the Teutonic shift of power and wealth from West to East is all but certain to continue as China is now the world's factory with a 1.4 billion people, and superior manpower that comes with it.

THE MORAL OF THE STORY

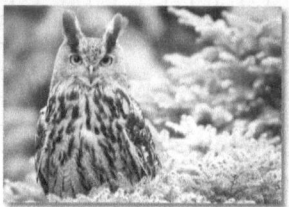

Only one thing in life is constant—change. Changes caused many civilizations, empires, and countries to rise, only to fall and disappear. Only knowledge, and skills can help someone to live and survive in such rapidly changing and competitive environments.

The same applies to the present civilization. Never before in the last 2,000 years has civilization faced such taxing demands on the planet's resources to sustain life as it exists today. Will the 21st century mark the end of current civilization?

---

[1] List of pre-modern great powers, en.wikipedia.org

ACKNOWLEDGEMENTS

☐ ☐ ☐

Many people directly or indirectly made many contributions to my books. But the biggest contributors, who made fundamental changes and altered the directions of my writing, were 2 men.

Dr. Samuel Oliner, who, after learning about my writing of 6 nonfiction books, encouraged me by all means to start with my short stories as the #1 priority (not #6, as I had planned before).

Harish Singhal, who, after reading about my life, became buoyant and excited because my life has been a real thriller. He impel to write about it. Enthusiastically, he gave me confidence that my books would become successful.

ILLUSTRATION CREDITS

□ □ □

Front cover illustration:
Vector Human Shape With Social Icons /graphicstock.com

Copyright page, back cover and spine: Sun symbol
SCA-Graphics/Dollar Photo Club

Short Story #1
Maksim Pasko/Dollar Photo Club

Short Story #2
a) Photoman/Dollar Photo Club
b) Skowron/Dollar Photo Club

Short Story #3.
a) Peter Zijlstra/Shutterstock
b) Valzan/Shutterstock

Short Story #4
Everett Historical/Shutterstock

Short Story #5
Syda Productions/Dollar Photo Club

Short Story #6
Vladgrin/Dollar Photo Club

Short Story #7
Marekuliasz/Shutterstock

Short Story #8
Aloksa/Dollar Photo Club

ILLUSTRATION CREDITS

Short Story #9
  Brocreative/Dollar Photo Club

Short Story #10
  NLPhotos/Dollar Photo Club

Short Story #11
  a) Tischenko Irina/Shutterstock
  b) Photoman29/Shutterstock

Short Story #12
  Kheng Guan Toh/Dollar Photo Club

Short Story #13
  a) Rook76/Shutterstock
  b) Everett Historical/Shutterstock

Short Story #14
  Robert Adrian Hillman/Shutterstock

Short Story #15
  Denis Belyaevskiy/Shutterstock

Short Story #16
  Art4all/Shutterstock

Short Story #17
  Sergey Peterman/Dollar Photo Club

Short Story #18
  Joanna Zielinska/Dollar Photo Club

Short Story #19
  Majivecka/Dollar Photo Club

Short Story #20
  Pinkcandy/Shutterstock

ILLUSTRATION CREDITS

Short Stories #1–#20
Eagle owl jurra8/Dollar Photo Club

Short Stories #1–#20. The Moral of the Story, Graph paper page, massimo_g

"The Forces of Innovations...Conflict?," an article by Carissa Giblin, *The Florida Engineering Journal*

THE AUTHOR'S, ALLA P. GAKUBA, BSCE, MAS, PhD, CONTRIBUTIONS TO ENGINEERING, TO NATIONAL WEALTH, AND TO WOMEN:

The Forces of Innovation…Conflict?
BY CARISSA GIBLIN, ARTICLE PROVIDED BY THE SOCIETY OF WOMEN ENGINEERS.
FLORIDA ENGINEERING JOURNAL, JANUARY 2004.

Many people ask Alla Gakuba how she innovates. She responds that she does not remember inventing something under normal circumstances; that is, without huge external and internal pressures. And it seems to be true. She came across a study while writing her dissertation for her PhD at George Washington University. The study surveyed thousands. of inventors asking them what factors were responsible for their innovations. The conclusion was great stress and pressure.

When Alla came to Baltimore, Maryland, in the beginning of the 1970s from the then USSR, she faced several environmental factors that created this pressure. There were few women engineers at the time. English was a new language to her. She knew only the metric system. Her husband was a physician working long hours, and they had two small children. It was the peak of the Cold War, and American engineers were paying close attention to Russian science and technology.

To her surprise, she was soon hired as a structural engineer. Never mind that Alla was not yet an engineer and that her English was only 4 months old. She had familiarized herself with the state building codes for a few days when the Chief Engineer told her her first project would be designing a three span bridge over a ramp—completely on her own.

He handed her a field drawing depicting the location of the ramp. As she took the drawing, dizziness overwhelmed her. "How in the world am I going to design it?" ran through her head. In her memory she went back to engineering school in expectation to retrieve some information about the design. She could recall none. In school she took math, physics, chemistry, static, kinematics, dynamics, strength of material, and reinforced concrete and steel. There was no trace of bridge design. She walked back to her office in despair.

On her way home that evening she stopped at the bridge site and examined the parapets, decks, piers, columns, and footings of the nearby ramps. The next day she had a lot of ideas on how to design the bridge. Looking at the field drawing of the ramp, she recognized that she needed to know the soil pressure under the bridge. Randomly, she sketched a dozen of soil borings.

When she gave her sketch to the soil department and asked for pressure measurements, they took her seriously and asked when she needed the information. She realized then she was on the right track. She started focusing on the bridge design. Alla decided to stay, and the pressure was on.

Alla was able to draw upon her engineering problem-solving skills and determination to succeed. She divided the bridge into separate structures. Using common sense and applying math, physics, and strength of materials, she designed each component one by one. All the pieces fit together as a puzzle, and it became the bridge. The company assembled a team of engineers to check her design and they were astounded at the calculations she used. She told them that no one gave her guidance so she invented each of the calculations.

Her design was accepted 100%. As they learned how simple it was, her calculation methods became standard in the company. Alla had created her own way of designing instead of copying the standard processes. Some time later, Alla learned bridge design traditionally involved a team of engineers each specializing in a particular structure. The company had given her the whole bridge to design to gain insight on Russian engineering and also to limit her success as the only female engineer in the company. In the end the company was so impressed, they started searching for another woman engineer.

Alla's next contribution involved an I-95, ten span bridge with four ramps over the Patapsco River in downtown Baltimore. She was given an opportunity to design this bridge alone. This time, the company trusted and believed in her; otherwise they would not have put all their eggs into one basket. And she lived up to their expectations. Not only did she design the bridge and ramps, but she also introduced a new foundation design. It required 30% less construction materials than standard foundations. The revolutionary aspect was that Alla's foundation designs took just one page of calculations for each pier.

Usually the design of foundation for each pier required computer programs followed by 70–80 pages of hand calculations. Her calculations and drawings were wrapped up and sent to an outside consulting company to check if they were correct.

Several months later, the consultants' hundreds of pages of computer printouts and calculations produced the same result as the innovations that Alla had calculated on one page.

Later, Alla was given a challenge to find a solution to a spiral design for 5.5 miles of aerial structure for the Baltimore Subway.

Only later did she learn that before approaching her, the company advertised in professional magazines across the country for engineers who could design a spiral for the subway. The company received no response. This was because no one had designed this before and no one wanted to risk their career.

So, Alla took on the project. She started with a blank piece of paper. The chief engineer told her about two French books about the new Paris subway sections housed in the Library of Congress in Washington, DC. She retrieved the books along with a French-English Civil Engineering dictionary. (She knew some French, but not civil engineering French.) The information only reinforced that what is applicable in Paris was not applicable in Baltimore. Also, the books were not about calculations and design of a spiral. Instead, they were about the philosophy, problems, and approach to design.

In the end, she made her own invention and found the solution for a spiral design. She calculated one span by long hand. Then, it was very simple to mirror her calculations and run the remaining 550 or so spans through the computer. The company wrote that Alla found the solution for spiral design of the aerial structure and that they considered it to be the most difficult engineering design. As for Alla, the spiral design was a nightmare that she cannot forget easily.

Alla cannot attribute the above contributions to herself only. She was a product of time, place, and circumstances. The time was the 1970s, which were the best technological years in her generation. The place was the US where equal employment opportunity laws were taking shape. She was a Russian in the US during the Cold War, where the great technological and political competitions for the dominance of the world were taking place between the two countries. She was given opportunity and responsibility and she lived up to their expectations. If Alla had stayed in the USSR, she doubts that she would have produced such contributions. In her opinion, there is no incentive to innovate in a familiar supportive environment. There must be a pressure.

Next, Alla managed the construction of the Baltimore Subway.

Her next objective was to enlarge her knowledge and became a better person. She received her Master's Degree from John Hopkins University where professors and students encouraged her to earn a PhD so she could become a role model for other women. She did. She received her Doctoral degree from George Washington University with a major in Management of Science, Technology, and Innovations. She was the first woman to graduate in this field. Her dissertation was ranked among the top 5% of the 250–300 dissertations which have been written in the last 15 years.

ARTICLE BY CARISSA GIBLIN

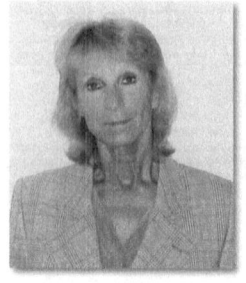 Alla Gakuba, PhD is a business analyst and consultant in Tampa, Florida. She earned her Bachelor of Science in Civil Engineering from Odessa Civil Engineering University in the former Soviet Union.

(Reprint of this article was granted by *The Florida Engineering Journal* on January 19, 2015.)

HAVE YOU READ? BOOKS BY
ALLA P. GAKUBA, BSCE, MAS, PhD

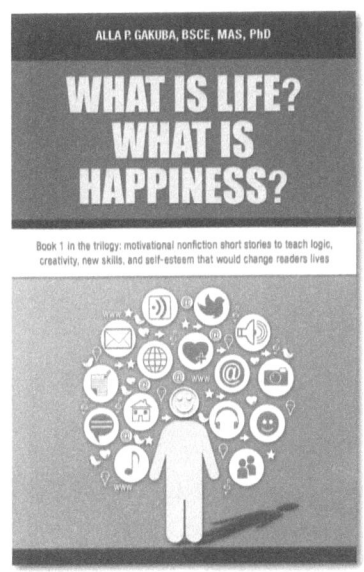
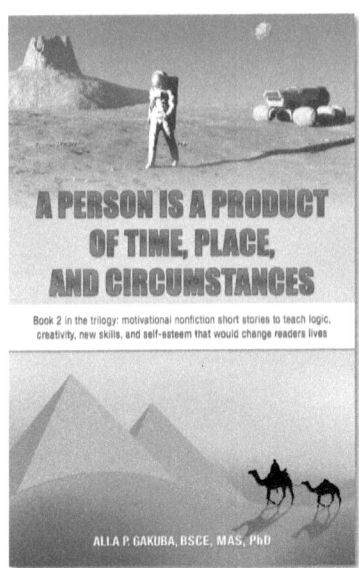
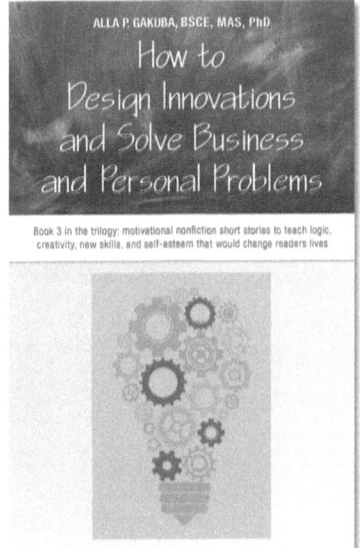

Available wherever books sold.

www.ingramcontent.com/pod-product-compliance
Lightning Source LLC
Chambersburg PA
CBHW021141080526
44588CB00008B/162

*9 7 8 1 9 4 3 1 3 1 0 0 6 *